THE FIRST-TIME MOM'S PREGNANCY HANDBOOK

THE FIRST-TIME MOM'S

PREGNANCY HANDBOOK

A WEEK-BY-WEEK GUIDE
from Conception through Baby's First 3 Months

By Bryn Huntpalmer

Illustrations by Abbie Winters

ROCKRIDGE
PRESS

Interior and Cover Designer: Julie Schrader
Art Producer: Sara Feinstein
Editor: Myryah Irby
Production Editor: Andrew Yackira
Illustrations © 2019 Abbie Winters. Author photo courtesy of © Heather Gallagher.

ISBN: Print 978-1-64152-854-2 | eBook 978-1-64152-855-9
RO

For Adelaide, Darwin, and Harvey
You make every day an adventure.

Contents

Foreword

IN MY CAREER as a primary care obstetrician, consultant, lecturer, author, and researcher, not a day goes by when I'm not exposed to pregnant women and their confusion. Misinformation, opinion, and skewed consent have replaced science, wisdom, and common sense. Where should a woman and her family turn when they are surrounded by so many unvetted resources and the hearsay and anecdotes of social media? So many books have been written about this subject that surfing Amazon can lead to even more confusion. And so many of these resources are based in fear and often lead to more questions than answers.

Pregnancy is a normal function of a woman's body that only rarely goes awry. When treated with confidence in this truth, this journey can and should be a time of joy and amazement. All too often, and unnecessarily, it is referred to as a medical problem that requires treatment. When pregnancy is looked at this way or when a woman is given a label of being "high risk," fear and anxiety replace joy. We now have generations of women whose experiences of pregnancy are tainted, and this is a cultural tragedy. We must find our way back to an understanding of the beauty and simplicity of nature's design.

In her new book, *The First-Time Mom's Pregnancy Handbook: A Week-by-Week Guide from Conception through Baby's First 3 Months,* author Bryn Huntpalmer gives us a roadmap to do just that. Knowledge is the key to overcoming fear and misinformation. Finding a compromise between oversimplicity and TMI in a pregnancy book can be a challenge. But, in *The First-Time Mom's Pregnancy Handbook,* Bryn has done just that. This book has a format that becomes familiar and is easy to read straight through. And the weekly descriptions, references, and suggested links make it easy to use as a resource, too.

Bryn is the mother of three and an entrepreneur, and admits to being a birth junkie! As the host of *The Birth Hour* podcast, she has listened to and learned from hundreds of women and shared the wisdom of actual experience. Not only does Bryn have the bona fides to offer her insight, she does so with a clarity and calmness that makes the journey from conception to three months postpartum encouraging rather than daunting. Straightforward rather than complicated. Safe rather than scary. Just what this doctor ordered!

—Stuart J. Fischbein, *MD FACOG*

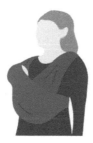

So, You're Gonna Be a Mom . . .

Congratulations, you're pregnant! Expecting a baby for the first time can bring on emotions you didn't even know you had, from excitement to full-on panic. To be honest, when I first saw that positive test, I was in disbelief, and then quickly transitioned into overdrive, feeling the need to do *all the things* right that moment. Naturally, I woke my husband before sunrise not only to share the news but also to run through a million scenarios and to-do lists. It might have been—I don't know—a bit much. But, hey, this a big deal, and it's completely normal to be having big emotions!

Once the initial joy and fear settled in, I read anything and everything I could find on pregnancy and childbirth. Between books, the internet, and unsolicited advice from friends, family, and even strangers, there is a lot of information out there! It can be really overwhelming and hard to know where to start. When I look back at my first pregnancy, I realize how much information overload I was suffering from.

Whether you're an over-researcher (like me) or feel completely clueless, this book will deliver essential information for your pregnancy and postpartum. Consider this your week-by-week action plan. This book will set up the next 12 months—yes, right into that infamous "fourth trimester"—so you can focus on the stuff that really matters, and be informed, empowered, and productive throughout your pregnancy and the first months of your baby's life.

The "Whys" and "Hows"

While no one can predict exactly what pregnancy will look like for you—I'll be the first to tell you that every single one is different—there are some key things to be aware of that will help you along the way and hopefully ease your concerns should the unexpected occur. So why should you take me with you on that journey? I'm a mother of three and the founder of *The Birth Hour*, a podcast that features women sharing uncensored pregnancy and birth stories of all types.

I've interviewed more than 400 women about their pregnancy and birth experiences. After all I learned and all I realized women wished they'd known, I teamed up with a childbirth educator, lactation consultant, and doula to create an online childbirth course called Know Your Options. In this course, we use an evidence-based approach to teach expecting couples everything they need to know to prepare for childbirth and life with a newborn. In writing this book, I've combined my own experience as a mom with what I've learned from being immersed in the world of pregnancy and birth over the last eight years. My hope is that you can feel educated every step of the way on what's happening, feel confident in your decision-making, and as a result, truly enjoy your pregnancy. We will also take a deep dive into how to prepare for and what to expect during the first three months of baby's life, also known as the "fourth trimester."

Information and Advice You Will Actually Use

While every pregnancy is unique, and each woman will encounter different symptoms and challenges, your body was made for this. Sometimes the amount of information we find in massive, encyclopedia-sized pregnancy books, not to mention Google, can be exhausting. In reality, women have been having babies for a lot longer than the internet has been around. While it's important to be informed about what's happening, try not to stress over every possible scenario or complication you hear or read about. The fact is, most pregnancies aren't, and shouldn't be, restrictive. Listening to your body and your intuition can go a long way in helping you focus on what applies to you and your baby.

There are plenty of things you *can* do during pregnancy, but not all that much that you *must* do. I want you to feel empowered to be an active participant in your care during pregnancy. Your care provider shouldn't be telling you what you can and can't do; they should have conversations with you that balance their medical expertise with your preferences and lived experience.

This book is your week-by-week guide to understanding what's happening to your body and how your baby is developing. I'll offer weekly goals for getting things done, from the medical stuff to taking care of yourself to preparing for baby. I've narrowed these down to the most relevant, need-to-know information for the majority of women and pregnancies. Keep in mind that not all appointments and goals will apply to everyone, or they may happen on a different timeline. Of course, if you ever have any concerns, whether or not they're covered in this book, please consult with your doctor or midwife.

What to Expect When ... Reading This Book

This book is divided into the three trimesters of pregnancy and the fourth trimester. The fourth trimester is the first 12 weeks of baby's life, when they are essentially a fetus outside the womb, relying on you for absolutely everything (no pressure, right?). To keep you organized, the book is further divided into months and then weeks. Each chapter will open with an action plan for that month and will be offered in this repeating format.

MONTHLY ACTION PLANS

Each month, I will provide you with a list of action-oriented goals based on your weekly milestone priorities and needs.

WEEKLY MILESTONES

Each week, I'll give you a rundown on your baby's development, symptoms you may be experiencing, any major appointments or events, and weekly goals you can focus on. These goals are categorized to make it easier to find the items that are most relevant to you at that time. Categories include:

+ **Call the Midwife:** Prenatal care and medical concerns.

+ **Symptoms 101:** Symptoms you may experience, though again, every woman is different. Many of these will also be covered in weekly "Mom Stats."

+ **Stay Strong:** Tips for focusing on your physical health.

+ **On the Menu:** Nutrition information and goals.

- **Birth Day:** Preparing for childbirth.

- **Rejuvenate:** Guidance for focusing on your emotional and mental health.

- **Make Room:** Home projects and baby preparation.

- **Budget Boot Camp:** Preparing your finances for baby.

- **Career Coach:** Navigating work while pregnant, plus preparing for maternity leave and beyond.

- **Gear Up:** Baby registry and gear information. We'll just discuss the basics.

- **This Is Love:** Tips for focusing on your relationship when two becomes three (or more!).

- **Decision Time:** Important decisions to consider during pregnancy and postpartum.

- **Postpartum Prep:** Preparing for your healing during the fourth trimester.

- **Baby Care:** Tips for taking care of your newborn.

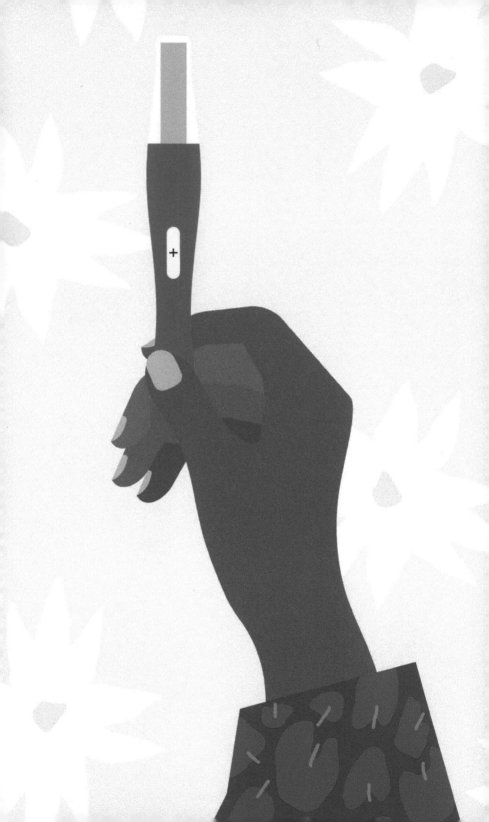

PART I

The First Trimester

Welcome to the first trimester! Once you've gotten that positive pregnancy test, you will likely start noticing some signs that your hormones are shifting, and your body is preparing to be your baby's home for the next nine months. Now is the time to make sure you are taking care of yourself by cutting out alcohol and tobacco, taking a prenatal vitamin, and eating a healthy diet.

One of the first things you'll likely wonder is when your baby will arrive. Your due date is calculated based on your last menstrual period (LMP). It will be 40 weeks from the first day of your LMP, so, when you find out you're pregnant, you've actually already snuck a few weeks of "pregnancy" in.

The first two months of your pregnancy are a bit of a waiting game. Unless you have a medical need to see your care provider early, you likely won't have your first appointment until you're about eight weeks. This is a great time to start thinking about the type of care provider you want (ob-gyn or midwife) and where you want to give birth (hospital, birth center, or at home). Choosing your care provider and where you give birth can be the most important decisions in determining how your birth will go. They should be made early, although you can change your mind at any time throughout your pregnancy.

The first trimester is often when you'll experience some of the most famous pregnancy symptoms: nausea, exhaustion, and sore breasts. We'll get into more specifics about these symptoms and others throughout this section, but keep in mind it is also completely normal to not experience any symptoms during early pregnancy.

Chapter 1

The First Month

The first month of pregnancy is when your body does the magic of conceiving. Whether you have been actively tracking your cycle or this is a surprise pregnancy, many things have to go right for your baby to come to be. If you're reading this book before getting pregnant, this chapter will cover tips to keep in mind.

Month 1 Action Plan:

- Evaluate your lifestyle: What are you putting into your body? Check your diet and exercise routine and be sure you're taking a prenatal vitamin.

- Fertility tips: If you're not already pregnant, start tracking your cycle. It can also be helpful to have ovulation and pregnancy tests on hand so you aren't making late-night runs to the store when you're desperate to know!

- It is completely normal for it to take a while to get pregnant, and most doctors won't be concerned until you've been trying for a year.

Week 1 Milestones

■ BABY'S STATS

+ Right now, your body is preparing your uterus for the next egg to be released—hopefully your baby.
+ You are born with all of the eggs you'll ever have, and it is possible to release two eggs in one month (fraternal twins).

■ MOM'S STATS

+ You're currently having your period, shedding your uterine lining in preparation for making a new lining for your baby.
+ You may be experiencing bloating, cramping, and hormonal shifts.

■ NOT-TO-MISS APPOINTMENTS

It's a great idea to get an annual exam before you start trying to conceive. Your doctor can suggest a prenatal vitamin, run any necessary blood work, and do a Pap smear if you're due for one. They can be uncomfortable during pregnancy, so better to get it out of the way!

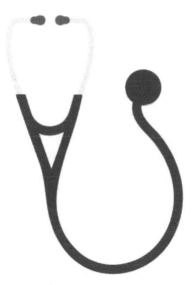

WEEK 1 GOALS

Gear Up Download a fertility-tracking app to document things like your temperature, cervical mucus—a.k.a. discharge—and any other symptoms that come up. A quality fertility app (I like Ovia) will help you predict your fertile window to increase your chances of getting pregnant.

Rejuvenate If you've been TTC (trying to conceive) for many months, getting your period can be hard. Try to practice some self-care, and visualize your body preparing for the next egg to be released—your baby!

KEY ADVICE

The amount of exercise that you are able to do during pregnancy is directly correlated to how much exercise you were doing before you got pregnant, so consider getting into a routine now. If you aren't already a frequenter of the gym, choose something you love and make it a habit. Swimming, yoga, and walking are great low-impact options.

Facing a Loss

Unfortunately, miscarriage is a necessary part of the discussion around pregnancy. Between 10 and 25 percent of recognized pregnancies end in miscarriage. Most miscarriages happen in the first few weeks, with the rate of miscarriage dropping to between 2 and 4 percent after week eight. By the end of the first trimester, the rate of miscarriage is less than 1 percent.

That being said, no number of facts or statistics will erase the way you feel after a loss. In all of the interviews I've done, I've found that everyone grieves their loss differently. I had a very early miscarriage and cried for days. I shared my experience on @thebirthhour Instagram account and received thousands of responses from women who had been exactly where I was.

If you miscarry in the first few weeks of pregnancy, it will likely happen on its own in the form of a heavier-than-normal period and cramping. Sometimes you'll need medical help to complete your miscarriage, and your care provider will discuss your options.

Most women physically recover very quickly from miscarriage and can begin trying to conceive the very next month. But it may take much longer to recover emotionally. Be gentle with yourself and reach out to friends or a professional for help processing what you've been through. There is also a supportive Instagram community (@ihadamiscarriage) run by a psychologist specializing in reproductive and maternal mental health. You are most definitely not alone.

■ BABY'S STATS

+ Your baby's egg is being released and hopefully will be fertilized by the sperm next week.
+ Fun fact: From the moment the sperm hits the egg, your baby's DNA and sex are set! Of course, it will be a while before you find out the sex of the baby and whether they got Mom's curly hair.

■ MOM'S STATS

+ Hopefully you've been tracking your cycle and are noticing signs of ovulation, like egg-white cervical mucus and a spike in your temperature.
+ Another great option is to use pee sticks that test for the luteinizing hormone (LH), the hormone released just before ovulation. Once you get a positive result, your egg should release within 24 to 48 hours.

■ NOT-TO-MISS APPOINTMENTS

You're only fertile for about six days a month, with the most fertile days being the day before and day of ovulation. It's recommended to have sex at least every other day around ovulation (days 12 to 16 of your cycle for most women).

WEEK 2 GOALS

This Is Love If you are trying to conceive naturally, that is, without the help of a donor or medical intervention such as in vitro fertilization (IVF), sex can become fairly mechanical, especially if you've been trying for more than a few months. Try to reconnect with your partner in order to make sex more enjoyable and less utilitarian. You can plan a romantic date night or even coordinate a fun trip around your fertile days.

Rejuvenate You hear it all the time: "As soon as I stopped stressing about getting pregnant, it happened." This is frustrating to hear when you're in the thick of trying to conceive (TTC), but it's worth keeping in mind and doing your best to find activities that lift some of the stress.

KEY ADVICE

Ovulation and pregnancy tests can get pricey! If you order test strips in bulk from Amazon, you can get them for a few cents each and save money. In a pinch, most dollar stores also carry pregnancy and ovulation tests, and Walmart has affordable store-brand options, as well.

■ BABY'S STATS

+ If your egg was fertilized, it is rapidly dividing cells, and it has a new name: blastocyst.
+ The blastocyst is preparing to travel through your fallopian tubes on its way to your uterus, where it will implant in your uterine wall.

■ MOM'S STATS

+ Your cervical mucus may be thickening and becoming more prevalent.
+ If you conceived, you likely won't have any symptoms yet. Although it can be tempting to search the internet after every little twinge you feel to see whether it's a pregnancy symptom, try to be patient.

■ NOT-TO-MISS APPOINTMENTS

Many women ovulate during this week, too, so it's a good idea to keep having sex, especially if you aren't tracking ovulation closely. Even if you are pretty sure you've already ovulated, it can be nice to have some no-pressure lovemaking for a change.

WEEK 3 GOALS

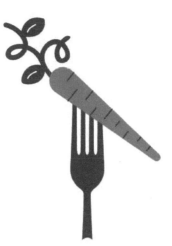

On the Menu This is a great time to look at your diet and make sure you're getting in your daily servings of veggies and plenty of protein. The first trimester can bring nausea and make it hard to eat anything other than bread, so try to frontload those nutrients now.

Stay Strong Now is the time to cut out tobacco and alcohol use. Many women ask about the occasional glass of wine, and you'll have to use your judgment there. I recommend the book *Expecting Better* by Emily Oster, which really dives into the research and evidence around the dos and don'ts of pregnancy.

KEY ADVICE

The level of the hormone human chorionic gonadotropin, commonly referred to as hCG or "the pregnancy hormone," is way too low to show up on a home pregnancy test until two weeks after you ovulated. You may be anxious to start testing, but save your money during what is known as the two-week wait. Test once the wait is up.

■ BABY'S STATS

+ Your baby is officially called an embryo and is itty-bitty—the size of a poppy seed!
+ The embryo is now securely implanted in the lining of your uterus and is developing a yolk sac that will nourish it until the placenta is formed.

■ MOM'S STATS

+ It's possible you could have some implantation bleeding toward the end of this week, which occurs when the egg implants in your uterine wall, but only about 30 percent of women get this early pregnancy sign.
+ You might be a little bloated, but it can be hard to tell whether it's pregnancy or your body preparing for your next period.

■ NOT-TO-MISS APPOINTMENTS

Time to take that pregnancy test! It's recommended to test first thing in the morning, because your urine is more concentrated with the pregnancy hormone at that time of day. If you're testing this week, you should be using an early result test that is sensitive enough to pick up smaller amounts of hCG.

WEEK 4 GOALS

Stay Strong Make sure you're taking a prenatal vitamin that contains 800–1000mg of methylated folate (L-Methylfolate). It's vital in the formation of your baby's neural tube, the first step in forming baby's nervous system.

Symptoms 101 The first trimester comes with a long list of symptoms thanks to big hormonal shifts. You may notice that your breasts are tender and maybe even getting bigger. Don't worry if you aren't experiencing any pregnancy symptoms yet—you might be one of the lucky women who sail through the first trimester symptom-free.

KEY ADVICE

Try to wait until later in the week to start testing. Most home pregnancy tests will give a correct result if you have already missed your period. Hopefully, you have those pregnancy test strips I mentioned and can test freely without spending a small fortune. It can become an obsession!

Chapter 2

The Second Month

Eek! You're pregnant! You've seen that positive pregnancy test, and your mind is racing over all of the to-dos before meeting your baby. Luckily, you have many months to figure it all out, and we are going to tackle everything one week at a time.

Month 2 Action Plan:

- Find a doctor or midwife and make your first appointment.
- Start exploring your options around childbirth; you'll want your preferences to align with those of the care provider you choose.
- Consider your lifestyle as you prepare for baby and discuss any potential changes (house, job, location, etc.) with your partner, if you have one.

Week 5 Milestones

■ BABY'S STATS

+ Baby is tiny now (the size of an apple seed), but baby grows rapidly during the first trimester and is hard at work, already developing organs.
+ You won't be able to hear a heartbeat for several weeks, and baby still looks more like a tadpole than a human.

■ MOM'S STATS

+ You may finally start to notice some symptoms of pregnancy during week 5. Common symptoms this week are sore breasts, cramping, nausea, and tiredness.
+ You won't have a visible belly until around week 12, but you may experience some bloating.

■ NOT-TO-MISS APPOINTMENTS

If you've already chosen a care provider, go ahead and give them a call to set up your first appointment. It likely won't be for a few weeks, but it's good to get on the schedule now. If you haven't chosen one yet, set up interviews ASAP.

WEEK 5 GOALS

Decision Time It's time to start interviewing doctors and/or midwives to see who is the best fit. If you have a partner, bring them with you to these appointments, because it will be important for them to feel comfortable with your care provider, as well. See lists of suggested questions to ask a midwife on page 18 and to ask an ob-gyn on page 39.

Call the Midwife If you choose to deliver with a midwife, most only take on a set number of births per month. So as soon as you find out you're pregnant, you'll want to make sure the midwife you've chosen is available. Ob-gyns typically have more flexibility, because they work in groups and aren't on call 24/7 around your due date.

It's a common misconception that midwives only attend out-of-hospital births. In fact, many ob-gyn practices work alongside midwives, and some midwives work at birth centers within the hospital. Outside of the United States, most women see midwives, and ob-gyns are only called in when a high-risk situation arises. Even if you know you want a hospital birth, I encourage you to meet with a midwife and ask questions about how her scope of practice is different from a doctor's.

Questions When Interviewing a Midwife

Do research on the midwifery model of care prior to meeting with midwives. Most will follow pretty similar practices around physiological birth, with some being more hands-on than others. Feeling comfortable and safe with your midwife and trusting them with your care is the most important thing. An initial interview as well as all regular prenatal appointments with your midwife will be about an hour long, so there is plenty of time to get all your questions answered. Here are some suggestions to have on hand during that initial interview. Highlight the ones that are important to you.

■ TRAINING AND EXPERIENCE

+ What license do you hold? How long have you been practicing, and how many births have you attended?
+ What are your fees? Do you offer payment plans or accept insurance?
+ Will you be available by phone or text, and what hours are you available?
+ How many planned births do you take on per month?
+ Who is your backup midwife in case you aren't available when I go into labor?
+ What equipment do you bring with you to a birth?
+ Do you have any apprentices or other support?
+ Are you backed by an ob-gyn?
+ What is your hospital transfer rate? What's the most common reason for transfer?
+ Which hospital would you recommend in case of transfer? Will you describe what past transfers have looked like for your patients?
+ What is your view on VBACs (vaginal birth after cesarean)? What is your success rate?
+ If my baby is breech, what is your protocol?
+ What is your experience with neonatal resuscitation?
+ What are the most common complications you encounter, and how are they handled?
+ Have you ever lost a baby or mother? If so, what happened?

■ SCREENINGS AND TESTS

+ Which screenings and tests do you recommend? Do you perform the tests, or would I go elsewhere?

+ Do you require a Group B strep test? What is the protocol if I am Group B positive? (For more info on Group B strep, see page 108.)
+ If I become "high risk," what is the process? What high-risk situations do you have experience with?

■ INTERVENTIONS

+ In labor, do you routinely perform cervical checks? Why or why not?
+ If my water breaks, do you put a time restriction on my labor?
+ What is your recommendation for a labor that stalls? Do you have a time limit on labor? Or the pushing phase?
+ What is your episiotomy rate? In what situations would you recommend an episiotomy?

■ LABOR SUPPORT

+ Do you support water birth? Do you have birth tubs available?
+ What other labor coping tools do you offer? (e.g., birth ball, rebozo, birth stool, essential oils, massage)
+ Will you support me or my partner in catching our own baby?

■ POSTPARTUM & NEWBORN CARE

+ What are your views on delayed cord clamping?
+ What postpartum and newborn care do you offer?
+ Do you offer newborn testing?

- If I deliver at a birth center, how long would I stay there afterward?
- Do you provide postpartum home visits?
- Do you offer breastfeeding support?

Again, listen to your gut when making your final decision. Since most midwives practice a similar model of care, personality might be one of the biggest factors in choosing a midwife. It's important that you trust and like your midwife.

Week 6 Milestones

■ BABY'S STATS

- Your baby is doubling in size each week and is now about the size of a pea.
- Baby still looks like a sea creature, but they are definitely visible on an ultrasound now, though you probably won't have your first scan until eight weeks.

■ MOM'S STATS

Your body is getting slammed with hormonal changes, and you may feel tired or moody as a result.

■ NOT-TO-MISS APPOINTMENTS

Unless you have a prior medical indication for an early ultrasound, you likely won't go in for another couple of weeks. If any concerns arise before your first appointment, always call your care provider right away.

WEEK 6 GOALS

This Is Love If you're feeling like you're going to throw up all the time or are actually throwing up, you may not be in the mood for sexy time. Your partner may be the one holding your hair back, which probably won't put them in the mood, either. Give yourself space to focus on feeling better, and know that for many couples, the second trimester is very hot and heavy.

On the Menu If your tummy is feeling queasy, it can be helpful to eat bland starchy foods like toast, macaroni and cheese, and mashed potatoes. Don't stress about your nutrition right now. Focus on keeping down anything you can, and make sure you're taking your prenatal vitamin.

KEY ADVICE

While cramping and spotting are common for many women, extreme pain is not. If you experience excruciating pain, it could be an ectopic pregnancy, which is most likely to occur between weeks 6 and 8. An ectopic pregnancy is when the fertilized egg implants in your fallopian tubes instead of your uterus, and it requires immediate medical care.

■ BABY'S STATS

+ Your baby is now the size of a blueberry and is growing fast! Vital parts like kidneys, the liver, and arm/leg buds are forming.
+ A large forehead is visible as the brain forms, making your sweet blueberry look a little like an alien.

■ MOM'S STATS

Even if you aren't actually throwing up, you might be experiencing occasional or consistent nausea or food aversions. Again, the hormone hCG is to blame. This usually subsides by the end of the first trimester.

■ NOT-TO-MISS APPOINTMENTS

If you have a partner, be sure to coordinate schedules when making your first prenatal appointment so they can be there. Many doctors will do an ultrasound at this appointment to confirm your due date, and your partner won't want to miss seeing your little bean for the first time.

WEEK 7 GOALS

Symptoms 101 You may experience constipation during pregnancy due to hormones that relax your muscles and slow things down. Drinking lots of water and eating plenty of fiber can help, but you'll definitely want to consult your care provider before taking any over-the-counter medications to treat constipation.

Birth Day Have you thought about the type of birth you want? Prepare a list of questions to ask your care provider at your first appointment to make sure you're on the same page. One tip: ask them what a typical birth looks like for them and pay attention to their response rather than asking whether they would be willing to accommodate a specific request you have. Odds are that they will follow their usual protocol when it comes to the big day.

Week 8 Milestones

■ BABY'S STATS

+ Your baby is a little more than 1 cm from head to bum—about the size of a raspberry.
+ Baby is developing ears, although hearing is a little way off.
+ The placenta is starting to take over providing nutrients to your baby as the yolk sac shrinks.

■ MOM'S STATS

You may be experiencing mixed feelings about your pregnancy, and that is totally normal. Your hormones are raging, your whole life is changing, and you're coping with some pretty gnarly symptoms.

■ NOT-TO-MISS APPOINTMENTS

This week or next is likely the week you've been waiting for! You finally have your first prenatal appointment and may even get to see your baby via ultrasound and hear the heartbeat. Dating ultrasounds are common at eight weeks, so if you are unsure of your last menstrual period (LMP) or conception date, be prepared for your estimated due date to shift slightly. You'll also be able to see whether you're having more than one baby at this point!

WEEK 8 GOALS

Rejuvenate If you're having mixed feelings about your pregnancy, it can be helpful to connect with other women. Whether you reach out to a friend or join an online forum or Facebook group, talk about what you're feeling. You aren't alone.

Career Coach Most women wait to tell their boss that they are pregnant until they start showing, but, if you are experiencing symptoms that are affecting your job performance and you feel comfortable sharing, it might be a good idea to let them know so they can better accommodate you. Let your employer know your news right away if you're working in an environment where you may be exposing the baby to toxins, like in a lab or around lots of chemicals or radiation.

Why Am I High Risk?

Hearing that you are having a "high-risk" pregnancy can be scary, but this label doesn't mean that there will be health problems for you or baby. It just means doctors will want to monitor you more closely for specific concerns throughout your pregnancy. You will be getting some extra attention from your care provider in the form of more appointments, scans, and testing. It also likely means that you will need to give birth in a hospital under the care of an ob-gyn.

A few common factors that contribute to being labeled high risk are:

+ advanced maternal age* (see note on page 27)
+ being over- or underweight** (see note on page 27)
+ family history of genetic disorders
+ pregnant with multiples
+ previous history with pregnancy loss

+ issues with your placenta or uterus
+ complications that arise during pregnancy
+ other medical conditions

We'll go over prenatal and genetic testing in more depth during weeks 10 and 15, but keep in mind that if you're high risk, you'll likely be offered more extensive (and possibly excessive) testing. A wonderful resource for women with high-risk pregnancies is Parijat Deshpande's book *Pregnancy Brain: A Mind-Body Approach to Stress Management during a High-Risk Pregnancy.*

*"Advanced maternal age" typically refers to women who are over the age of 35, though not everyone agrees on the exact age, or how helpful this label is. Most older moms have normal pregnancies and healthy babies.

**Being overweight shouldn't automatically make you high risk. If you notice a bias from your care provider solely related to your size, look for another provider. Resources are available at plussizebirth.com and sizefriendly.com.

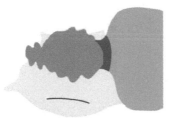

Chapter 3

The Third Month

It's finally time to start checking in on baby by getting some routine tests done. In this chapter, we'll go over all the first-trimester screenings and lab work you can expect.

Month 3 Action Plan:

- Go in for your first prenatal appointment and decide which tests you want and which ones you'd rather skip.
- Baby is starting to look like a human, and, with your first ultrasound picture printed out, if you're comfortable, it may be time to share your news with friends and family!

Week 9 Milestones

■ BABY'S STATS

+ Baby weighs around .07 ounce and is about the size of a cherry.
+ No longer referred to as an embryo, your baby is now a fetus.

■ MOM'S STATS

You may be still in the thick of first-trimester nausea and exhaustion and may be experiencing a couple of other symptoms, like congestion and headaches. Just like everything else, these are caused by hormonal changes. Your body should adjust to these hormones by the end of month 3.

■ NOT-TO-MISS APPOINTMENTS

Your doctor or midwife will need to run blood work and collect a urine sample in order to establish a baseline to keep an eye out for complications during pregnancy, including things like anemia, preeclampsia, and gestational diabetes.

WEEK 9 GOALS

Call the Midwife Your care provider needs to know your blood type and Rh status. Rhesus (Rh) is a protein found in most people's blood (Rh positive); however, some people are missing this protein (Rh negative). If you are Rh negative and your baby is Rh positive, and if your blood mixes with baby's, your body may start to produce antibodies that will attack the baby's blood. If you are Rh negative, you will be offered a Rhogam shot at 28 weeks that keeps your body from making those antibodies.

Budget Boot Camp It's never too early to start planning for things like paying for your prenatal care or even childcare once baby arrives. Sit down and take stock of your monthly income and expenses.

KEY ADVICE

Start a journal to document milestones, symptoms, and feelings about your pregnancy. Not only is this a cathartic activity, it actually comes in handy for future pregnancies when you're trying to remember things like when your energy levels increased or how big your baby measured at that first appointment.

■ BABY'S STATS

+ Baby is a little over an inch long now, around the size of a prune, and weighs about .14 ounce.

+ All of baby's vital organs are formed and starting to function, and baby is even growing hair and nails.

■ MOM'S STATS

You might start noticing a little baby bump, especially after a big meal! Some growing pains can come along with that. Round-ligament pain, which feels like sharp shooting pains on the underside of your belly, is common throughout pregnancy and can start as early as 10 weeks.

■ NOT-TO-MISS APPOINTMENTS

Around week 10, you will be offered some screenings and genetic tests. The most common is the nuchal translucency screening (NT scan), which is performed via ultrasound and measures the amount of fluid at the base of your baby's neck. This can identify the potential risk of chromosomal abnormalities, such as Down syndrome.

WEEK 10 GOALS

Decision Time Between 10 and 13 weeks, there are a few decisions to make about screening for genetic disorders. There is a blood test offered that has a few different names, including Verifi, Harmony prenatal test, and MaterniT21. It determines the risk of chromosomal abnormalities like Down syndrome or trisomy 13 and is reported to be between 91 and 99 percent accurate. This test can also tell you the sex of your baby if you want to find out!

This Is Love Talk to your partner about these tests. Hearing all the potential things that could go wrong can be anxiety-producing for them, too.

> **KEY ADVICE**
>
> *Optional genetic screenings aren't always covered by insurance, so you'll want to check with your care provider or health insurance to make sure you aren't going to incur major out-of-pocket costs by electing to get these tests.*

Week 11 Milestones

■ BABY'S STATS

+ Baby is 1.5 inches long and weighs .25 ounce, about the size of a strawberry.
+ Your baby has 10 tiny fingers and 10 tiny toes and is looking more and more like a baby, although their head still accounts for half of their body weight.

■ MOM'S STATS

Even if you can't quite see a true baby bump yet, your jeans might be getting a little tighter as your belly grows and your appetite increases.

■ NOT-TO-MISS APPOINTMENTS

If you're feeling less exhaustion, now is a great time to get back into (or start) a regular exercise habit. Prenatal yoga is an excellent, gentle exercise that can help prepare your body for giving birth. See whether you can try a free class at your local yoga studio.

WEEK 11 GOALS

Stay Strong Walking every day is fantastic preparation for giving birth. My midwife recommended between two and five miles a day, though getting any steps in helps. If you have the time, put in your earbuds, put on a great podcast (I'm partial to *The Birth Hour* for birth prep!), and walk, walk, walk.

On the Menu If your appetite is back, try to make healthy choices. Protein is good for baby's brain development. Aim for 75 to 100g of protein each day. And be sure to eat lots of iron-rich vegetables like leafy greens, which will help prevent pregnancy-induced anemia.

KEY ADVICE

Pants getting a bit snug? If you aren't quite ready to invest in maternity clothes, use a hair tie or rubber band through the loop of your jeans to give you a couple of extra inches. Belly bands, stretchy fabric tubes, can also turn most pants into makeshift maternity pants.

■ BABY'S STATS

+ Baby is about 2 inches long and weighs 0.5 ounce, around the size of a lime.
+ Most of your baby's main organs have formed, along with all their functions, and the rest of gestation is all about growing and developing to be able to live outside the womb.

■ MOM'S STATS

You may develop a new symptom around this time: dizziness. The increased blood flow to your baby can cause light-headedness or dizzy spells.

■ NOT-TO-MISS APPOINTMENTS

This week will likely include your second prenatal appointment. You'll have one appointment every four weeks up until you're 28 weeks pregnant. At these regular appointments, your doctor or midwife will test your urine, measure your belly, and listen to the baby's heartbeat.

WEEK 12 GOALS

Call the Midwife Bring any questions that have come up during the first trimester to your appointment this week. If you're seeing a midwife, your visit may be around an hour long. If you're seeing a doctor, you will likely have a shorter visit, so write down questions ahead of time to make sure you get them answered. See pages 18 and 39 for lists of potential questions.

Gear Up Your baby bump may be ready for some maternity clothes this week! Get a comfy pair of maternity leggings and some stretchy tank tops to start. These two items can be layered and paired with a variety of non-maternity clothes (think jackets, cardigans, and kimonos).

KEY ADVICE

The first signs of a linea nigra (a dark line down the middle of your belly) might start to appear this week. No worries—it's completely normal and will fade after pregnancy. It is also normal not to have a line at all.

Week 13 Milestones

■ BABY'S STATS

+ Baby is almost 3 inches long, weighs about .80 ounce, and is around the size of a lemon.
+ Baby's head accounts for one third of their body, and baby's eyes have formed, though they will remain fused shut until about 28 weeks.

■ MOM'S STATS

As any lingering nausea eases up, it may be swapped for heartburn. Heartburn is caused by pregnancy hormones relaxing the valve of your esophagus, which allows stomach acid to escape. This usually begins in the second trimester and can last through the rest of pregnancy.

■ NOT-TO-MISS APPOINTMENTS

Many expecting moms decide to share their pregnancy news with friends and family around this time. It can start to make this baby thing a lot more real. One tip: Don't share your exact due date. This way, if you go past 40 weeks, people won't bug you every day until baby arrives.

WEEK 13 GOALS

Rejuvenate Don't stress about being stressed. You have a lot going on, and a certain amount of stress and anxiety is expected. Everyone will tell you stress isn't good for the baby, which can make you even more stressed out. Give your-self space to feel what you're feeling, and reach out for help if needed.

Career Coach If you sit at a desk for most of the day, try to get up and move around every hour. It may also be a good idea to request accommodations like a standing desk or an exercise ball to sit on.

KEY ADVICE

There are a few ways to ease heartburn: eat several small meals a day; don't drink with your meals; and avoid spicy and fatty foods, caffeine, chocolate, and alcohol. If your heartburn is severe, your doctor can prescribe medica-tion. Papaya enzyme pills, which can be found at any drugstore, also may help.

What to Consider When Interviewing an Ob-gyn

When it comes to specific questions, I recommend focusing on the things that matter to you most and letting them elaborate on their own so you get a feel for their normal procedures. If you'd like to explore more potential questions, go to thebirthhour.com.

■ THINGS TO KEEP IN MIND

+ Play dumb. Don't bring in your birth plan and say, "This is what I want. Do you do this?" It's a good idea to find out how they normally practice, since it's likely that they will treat your birth the same way.
+ Ask around. Ask childbirth educators, doulas, and moms in your area. The International Cesarean Awareness Network (ICAN) is a great resource. Find your local ICAN chapter at ican-online.org.
+ Be confident. Your care provider is a member of YOUR birth team. You have the right to ask questions and expect answers.
+ Have a list of questions, prioritized according to what you most want to know. It will likely be a short appointment, and you want to make sure you get your most important questions answered.

■ QUESTIONS TO ASK

+ If I have a question between appointments, will I be able to reach you? Who will be available to answer questions outside normal business hours?
+ What typically happens when one of your patients goes into labor?
+ What are your thoughts on VBAC (vaginal birth after cesarean)? If this is your first baby, this obviously doesn't apply to you, but it's a good indicator of how supportive they are of patients' birth preferences in general.
+ How many days past my estimated due date are you comfortable with me going?

+ When would you recommend an induction? An episiotomy? A cesarean?

  • *If they say, "When medically necessary," then ask, "When is that, exactly?"*
  • *What are your rates at which these interventions are performed?*

+ How are decisions made during labor? Under what circumstances would you say I don't get to make decisions? (The answer should be "Never." See more about informed consent on page 95.)
+ What's your view on delayed cord clamping?

■ POTENTIAL RED FLAGS

+ Rolls eyes, dismisses your questions, doesn't take time to relate to your concerns.
+ Doesn't treat you like a team member or a competent, intelligent person in charge of your own body.
+ Predicts your baby will be too big.
+ Says VBAC is not an option (or is strongly discouraged).
+ Doesn't know their own statistics (e.g., rate of cesareans or inductions) or not willing to share.

Trust your instincts and judgment. What was your impression of the doctor? If you have a partner, how did they feel? Good signs would be feelings of connection, excitement, and trust. If you feel anxious or uncertain, interview more doctors. The right fit for you is out there!

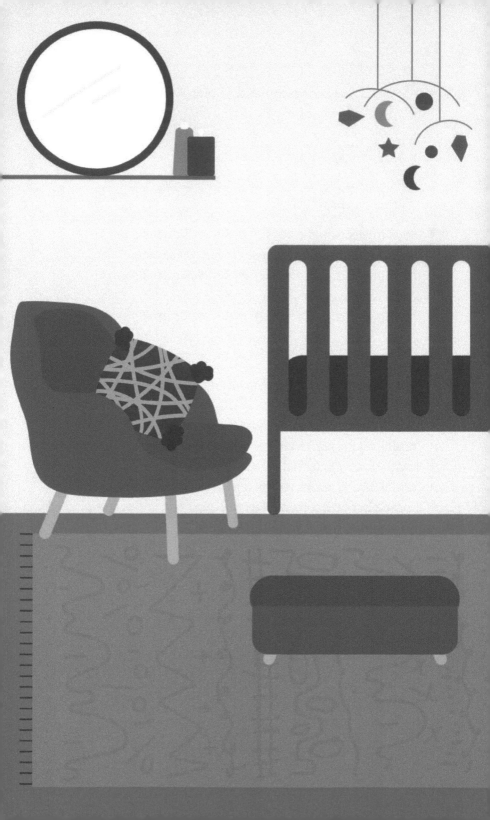

PART II

The Second Trimester

Welcome to the second trimester! For many women, this is considered the honeymoon trimester. Those early pregnancy symptoms are easing up, and your belly isn't so big that you can't pick things up off the ground. Enjoy this time and plan fun things like date nights, sleeping in, and even a babymoon (one last vacation as a couple before baby arrives). Use these weeks to do things like work on the nursery, choose a childbirth class, and prepare for maternity and/or paternity leave.

You'll have some big appointments this month, including the anatomy scan, which is performed via ultrasound. During this scan, your baby will get a full in utero physical, and you'll have the opportunity to learn baby's sex. Your provider will also be looking at your placenta to make sure it's in an optimal position for birth. You'll be offered more genetic screenings during the second trimester, especially if anything was abnormal on your first-trimester screenings. Finally, your doctor or midwife will order a complete blood count test, which is a simple blood draw. This is compared to your baseline blood work from the beginning of pregnancy to alert your provider to any concerns.

It's also never too early to start thinking about your birth. Get on the same page with your partner regarding who'll be notified when you go into labor and whether you want anyone else at your birth. Your parents may ask, so it's good to be in agreement before the requests start coming in. Also, if you plan to, now's a great time to start interviewing doulas. A birth doula is someone trained to provide emotional, physical, and informational support during your labor. A postpartum doula comes to your house to help take care of you and baby during the day or overnight.

Chapter 4

The Fourth Month

The first month of the second trimester should bring some relief from early pregnancy symptoms. This is the perfect time to check some baby prep items off your to-do list.

Month 4 Action Plan:

- As your hormone levels balance out, take advantage of your newfound energy and get out of the house—exercise is amazing for you and baby.

- Start a baby registry and nail down a date for your baby shower if you're planning to have one. See page 48 for suggestions about what to include on your registry!

Week 14 Milestones

■ BABY'S STATS

+ Baby is about 3.5 inches long, weighs 1.5 ounces, and is around the size of a peach.
+ Baby is growing peach fuzz, called lanugo, and is learning to make facial expressions.

■ MOM'S STATS

Many women experience an increase in energy this week. Your baby bump is getting bigger, and it may start to attract well-meaning smiles from strangers.

■ NOT-TO-MISS APPOINTMENTS

Get your baby shower on the calendar if you are having one. Most moms like to plan a baby shower for sometime between 28 and 34 weeks. It can also be fun to plan a "meet the baby" party for a couple of months after baby arrives. And it's completely fine to skip the baby shower altogether if you feel it may add to your stress.

WEEK 14 GOALS

Gear Up Time to start building your registry! Most baby registries are online now, so you don't even have to get out of your pajamas. My favorite online registry is Babylist—it's a universal registry that allows you to pull items from any store. Babylist also offers up-to-date shopping guides and sample registries.

Postpartum Prep Another great thing about Babylist is that you can add helpful things like home-cooked meals or dog walking for once baby is born. Alternatively, you could start a fund for a postpartum doula, probably one of the greatest gifts, especially if you don't have family nearby.

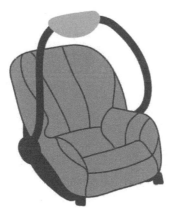

Creating your registry should be fun, not overwhelming. There are hundreds of different options for each category, and tons of items that are irresistibly cute or will make your life easier. So build your dream registry! Do keep in mind that every baby is different. I guess what I'm saying is, keep the receipts.

Baby Registry Basics

+ Car seat
+ Diapers and wipes
+ 10 outfits (infant gowns, sleepers, or onesies depending on the season)
+ 10 prefold cloth diapers to use as burp cloths
+ Safe place for baby to sleep
+ Swaddles
+ Pacifier (register for a few different types to see what baby prefers)
+ Baby seat or portable bassinet (a safe, convenient place to put baby while you take a shower or use the bathroom)
+ Front baby carrier, wrap, or sling
+ Thermometer
+ Baby nail clippers or file
+ NoseFrida Snot Sucker

- If bottle-feeding: bottles and bottle brush
- If breastfeeding: Order a pump for free through insurance, using a site like aeroflowbreastpumps.com
- Comfy robe and pajamas for you

Find more detailed lists on thebirthhour.com.

Week 15 Milestones

■ BABY'S STATS

- Baby is about 4 inches long, weighs 2.5 ounces, and is around the size of a pear.
- Baby's ears and eyes have moved to the proper places on baby's face and are growing rapidly.

■ MOM'S STATS

Your breasts are likely still growing, and you may even start to notice a little colostrum (baby's first food) leaking.

■ NOT-TO-MISS APPOINTMENTS

If you do further genetic screening, you'll have blood drawn sometime in the next four weeks. This test has a few different names, including quad screen, triple screen, AFP Plus, and multiple marker screening. Your doctor will speak with you about which test is right for you. Keep in mind these are not diagnostic tests; they can only determine your baby's risk for chromosomal abnormalities and can be indicators for possible further testing.

WEEK 15 GOALS

Career Coach If you haven't told your boss yet, now is probably the time. Schedule an in-person meeting and be straightforward. Let them know when you're due, when you plan to start maternity leave, and when you expect to return from maternity leave.

Stay Strong If you come down with a cold, suffer from allergies, or get a stomach bug, it can be hard to know which medications are safe to take, so ask your care provider. Another helpful resource is mothertobaby.org, which has fact sheets on over-the-counter and prescription drugs with a handy search function.

KEY ADVICE

If your breasts are significantly larger, it's time to get a bra that fits properly. You may want to opt for an inexpensive option, because your breasts are likely to continue to grow. Kindred Bravely makes supportive yet stretchy bras for moms of all sizes. Another great tip is to buy a bra extender.

■ BABY'S STATS

+ Baby is about 4.5 inches long, weighs 3.5 ounces, and is around the size of an avocado.
+ If you were to have an ultrasound this week, you might be able to see baby hiccuping or sucking their thumb.

■ MOM'S STATS

Many women experience leg cramps, or charley horses, during the second and third trimesters. They most often occur in the middle of the night.

■ NOT-TO-MISS APPOINTMENTS

You should have your second prenatal appointment around this week. Your care provider will check in on baby's size, and you will get to hear baby's heartbeat. You'll also schedule your anatomy scan, where baby will get a full-body checkup, for around 18 to 20 weeks.

WEEK 16 GOALS

On the Menu As your baby gets bigger, your body needs more nutrients to help baby grow. Hard-boiled eggs or a protein drink are an easy way to get a protein boost early in the day. There is even a brand called Baby Booster that tailors its ingredients specifically to pregnant women.

This Is Love For many women, sex drive returns in a big way during the second trimester. Unless you have a medical condition that has landed you on pelvic floor rest, sex is completely safe during pregnancy, so enjoy this newfound libido if you've got it.

KEY ADVICE

Need to decrease the occurrence and ease the pain of leg cramps? Try drinking lots of water before bed and taking a magnesium supplement. If you do wake up to leg cramps, try massaging and stretching your legs, and if that doesn't work, soak in a warm (but not hot) bath.

Week 17 Milestones

■ BABY'S STATS

+ Baby is about 5 inches long, weighs 5 ounces, and is the size of an onion.
+ Baby's ears are almost fully formed and can hear sounds through your belly.
+ Baby is also sensitive to light, even though their eyes are still fused shut.

■ MOM'S STATS

+ Your belly continues to grow. Recommended weight gain is one to two pounds a week during the second trimester, but don't stress if you're gaining a bit more or less.
+ Bleeding gums caused by pregnancy gingivitis can occur around this point. Caused by hormonal changes that make your gums inflamed and more susceptible to the bacteria in plaque, this symptom typically resolves quickly after baby is born.

■ NOT-TO-MISS APPOINTMENTS

Speaking of your gums, you should see your dentist during pregnancy for at least one checkup. Let them know you are pregnant so they can advise you about any symptoms you're experiencing and skip the X-rays.

WEEK 17 GOALS

Decision Time Look into your childcare options. It might seem crazy to be thinking about this, but, in some areas, day cares fill up fast. If you're planning to return to work, it's time to start touring day care centers or interviewing nannies so you can get on any waiting lists.

This Is Love Plan a babymoon! Whether it's an extravagant tour of Europe or a long weekend nearby, having something to look forward to as one last memorable trip with your partner is so fun. Since it's not recommended to fly after 36 weeks, the second trimester Is the perfect time for your babymoon.

Low-impact exercise is recommended because your joints and ligaments are looser due to relaxin (a pregnancy hormone), and your center of gravity is changing. Prenatal yoga, walking, and swimming are excellent choices. If you were already participating in a high-impact sport before pregnancy, it's usually okay to continue, but talk to your care provider to be sure.

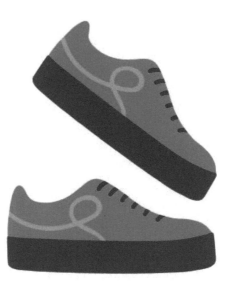

Chapter 5

The Fifth Month

This month is a big one! You'll pass the halfway mark of your pregnancy, and you'll have the opportunity to find out the sex of your baby.

Month 5 Action Plan:

- If you decide to have a doula, settle on one this month.
- Choose a childbirth class.
- Schedule your anatomy scan and decide whether you want to know the sex of the baby.

Week 18 Milestones

■ BABY'S STATS

+ Baby is about 5.5 inches long, weighs 6 ounces, and is around the size of a sweet potato.
+ Baby is practicing sucking and swallowing amniotic fluid in preparation for feeding after baby is born.
+ Baby's fingerprints are forming.

■ MOM'S STATS

You may start to notice varicose veins, typically on your legs and feet. They're caused by hormones opening up the veins, along with your uterus putting pressure on a major vein, called the vena cava, that circulates blood from your heart to your legs.

■ NOT-TO-MISS APPOINTMENTS

If you opted for the second-trimester genetic screening and something of concern came back, you might be offered an amniocentesis diagnostic test, which can diagnose a genetic disease in your baby. A needle is inserted into your belly to sample your amniotic fluid, then the chromosomes are analyzed in a lab.

WEEK 18 GOALS

On the Menu Pay attention to the amount of calcium and fiber in your diet. Calcium builds your baby's bones and teeth and keeps your own bones strong during pregnancy (aim for 1000mg a day). Fiber helps you avoid constipation (aim for 25 to 30g a day).

Rejuvenate There are many stressors when you're growing a human; it's important to take time to replenish your mind and connect with baby. Guided meditation is a great way to do that. Expectful is an app specifically for expecting and new mothers that focuses on helping you reduce stress, improve sleep, and connect with baby.

KEY ADVICE

Your blood volume increases by 50 percent during pregnancy, and iron is necessary for building your blood supply. You should always check with your doctor before taking any supplements or changing your diet while pregnant, but eating iron-rich foods and taking an iron supplement can be a solution. Unfortunately, traditional iron supplements can cause constipation, so look for a vegetable-based iron supplement like Floradix or MegaFood Blood Builder.

■ BABY'S STATS

+ Baby is about 6 inches long, weighs 8 ounces, and is around the size of a mango.
+ Baby's skin is covered in vernix, a cheesy coating that protects baby's skin in utero and may still be present at birth.

■ MOM'S STATS

You may start to feel baby's movements around this time. The first movements are called "quickening" and are like little flutters that can be difficult to distinguish from stomach gas.

■ NOT-TO-MISS APPOINTMENTS

This week or next is when you'll typically have your anatomy scan. Call ahead and ask whether there are any specific instructions for the day-of. Sometimes they'll want you to have a full bladder, and many moms swear by drinking a glass of juice right beforehand to get baby moving.

WEEK 19 GOALS

Budget Boot Camp Call your health insurance company for an estimate of your out-of-pocket expenses for your birth. While you're on the phone, also ask about the process for getting your baby added to the policy.

On the Menu Make sure you're staying hydrated. Drinking 10 to 12 eight-ounce glasses of water a day will help prevent constipation and is super important for keeping baby healthy. Dehydration can cause a reduction in amniotic fluid and has been connected to preterm labor. A large travel cup with a straw will help you drink more water.

KEY ADVICE

As your uterus gets bigger and heavier, it puts pressure on the vena cava (that large vein that carries blood to your lower half). Doctors recommend pregnant women sleep on their left side to prevent this. It's fine to switch to your right side, but try to avoid sleeping on your back.

■ BABY'S STATS

+ Baby is about 6.5 inches long, weighs 10 ounces, and is around the size of a bell pepper.
+ Baby is growing fingernails.
+ Baby is developing more regular sleep cycles and can be awakened by sound.
+ Baby's genitalia are formed, and an ultrasound can indicate the sex of the baby.

■ MOM'S STATS

Your feet may be swelling, especially if you live in a warm climate. Mild swelling is expected and is caused by weight gain, fluid retention, and/or the relaxin hormone spreading the ligaments in your feet. If you're experiencing extreme swelling, especially accompanied by headaches or dizziness, call your care provider immediately.

■ NOT-TO-MISS APPOINTMENTS

This week is the anatomy scan! This ultrasound takes 30 minutes to an hour. The technician will be trying to get images of all different angles of your baby's major organs and bones. Never hesitate to ask questions if you have any. You'll also have the option to find out baby's sex.

WEEK 20 GOALS

Career Coach Consult with Human Resources about your options around extended leave and the use of the FMLA (Family and Medical Leave Act). The FMLA requires larger companies to allow up to 12 weeks of unpaid leave for a serious health condition, and giving birth falls under this umbrella. You must request FMLA leave at least 30 days before taking it.

Decision Time Did you find out baby's sex? Now you get to decide whether to share it with friends and family. If you do, be prepared for an influx of gender-specific baby gifts you may not want to reuse with a sibling of the opposite sex.

KEY ADVICE

If you're not happy with your care provider, it's never too late to change. But some care providers won't take new patients after 20 weeks. When interviewing a replacement, be sure to address your concerns and gauge their response so you don't end up in the same situation twice.

What Is Preeclampsia?

Preeclampsia is a pregnancy-related condition in which your blood pressure spikes and your organs (usually liver and kidneys) begin to fail. Common symptoms include high blood pressure, swelling of your hands and face, protein in your urine, problems with your vision, dizziness, and severe headaches. Women at higher risk for preeclampsia include women under the age of 20 and over the age of 40, a previous history of preeclampsia, a mother or sister who had preeclampsia, first pregnancies, carrying multiples, and women with a BMI over 30.

Unfortunately, the only way to cure preeclampsia is by delivering the baby. Being diagnosed with preeclampsia before your baby is fully developed means that your doctor will have to do everything they can to keep your blood pressure down and buy as much time as possible for baby to develop. You might be prescribed bed rest as well as blood pressure medicine. You may also be given a steroid shot to help with the development of baby's lungs if they are born prematurely.

Preeclampsia typically occurs after 20 weeks, and your doctor or midwife will be on the lookout for warning signs of preeclampsia at your regular checkups. If you experience any severe headaches or blurriness of vision, contact your care provider immediately.

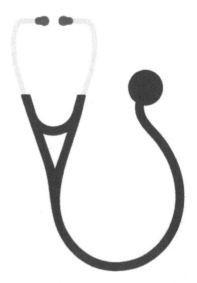

■ BABY'S STATS

+ Baby is 10.5 inches long, weighs 12 ounces, and is about the size of a banana.
+ The leap in growth is due to switching from measuring from head to bum to measuring from head to heel.
+ Your baby's arms and legs are in proportion to their body now, and baby's movements are more coordinated.

■ MOM'S STATS

You are most likely feeling baby's movements now and may be experiencing symptoms of your growing belly, like backaches, hip pain, or round-ligament pain.

■ NOT-TO-MISS APPOINTMENTS

Studies have shown mothers who have doulas at their births have lower rates of epidurals, cesareans, Pitocin, and the use of forceps or vacuum assistance. You can find one at Meet the Doula events, where you can meet with a bunch of doulas in the area, doulamatch.net, or dona.org, or, if you're on a tight budget, some hospitals have volunteer doula programs.

WEEK 21 GOALS

Decision Time Look into life insurance and talk to your partner about making a will. It's not the most fun thing to discuss, but you are likely to put it off further after baby is born.

Birth Day There are lots of options for in-person childbirth classes, including Lamaze, Bradley Method, Hypnobirthing, and Birthing from Within. You can also take an online class. At *The Birth Hour*, we created an evidence-based online course called Know Your Options that addresses all types of childbirth and takes you through postpartum and breastfeeding. You can find it at thebirthhour.com.

KEY ADVICE

Many women, even those who normally have clear skin, will experience acne during pregnancy. This can be frustrating, since you're limited in what medications you can use. Natural remedies, including witch hazel or essential oils (like frankincense and tea tree), offer skin support. (Check the Resources section on page 171 for a link to my blog on which essential oils are safe to use during pregnancy.) You might also try cutting out dairy and refined sugar.

■ BABY'S STATS

+ Baby is about 11 inches long, weighs 15.5 ounces, and is around the size of a papaya.
+ Baby is making facial expressions and reacting to sound.
+ Baby now has eyebrows, and baby's tear ducts are forming.

■ MOM'S STATS

You may start to notice Braxton-Hicks contractions. These are practice contractions that are not painful, but they can be surprising! Your entire stomach will get hard as your uterus tightens and releases. They won't come in any sort of pattern like the real-deal contractions will.

■ NOT-TO-MISS APPOINTMENTS

If you plan to have maternity photos taken, schedule them for between 30 and 34 weeks. Your bump is big enough to be the star of the photos, but you aren't so big that you're overly uncomfortable. If you're on a budget, consider asking a friend who's good with a camera.

WEEK 22 GOALS

Decision Time Consider whether you want to invest in cord blood banking or donating cord blood. Stem cells from your baby's umbilical cord blood can be preserved and stored in a blood bank. These are used to treat leukemia and other life-threatening diseases. Several companies offer this service, so, if you're interested, you should get a few cost breakdowns. Many hospitals also offer the option to donate cord blood that could be used to save another life. Find more info at bethematch.org.

Stay Strong Incorporate mini stretch routines throughout your day. Two stretches that are great for preparing your muscles for childbirth are squats and lunges.

KEY ADVICE

Listen to your body when you feel tired; choose sleep over a night out or another episode of your latest Netflix binge. Leave your phone in another room, get a good eye mask and earplugs, and sleep on the side of the bed closest to the bathroom for those middle-of-the-night pee breaks.

Birth Options and Preferences

This is meant to be a guide for exploring your options and then discussing them with your care provider. This is mostly tailored for hospital births but will apply to birth-center births in many areas, as well. If you bring a birth plan to the hospital, make it as brief as possible and label it "Birth Preferences," because—remember—birth rarely goes completely according to *plan*, and your preferences may change as labor progresses. Find more info on birth preferences for a home birth at thebirthhour.com.

■ LABOR & DELIVERY

+ What support people do you want in the labor room and when? Is there anyone who is not welcome?
+ Are you okay with medical students or residents in your labor room?
+ Do you want pain relief discussed right away or only if you ask for it?
+ Do you want to walk around and move during labor, including the option of using the shower or tub?
+ Do you want to self-hydrate (with a saline lock in case IV hydration is needed)?
+ Do you want to limit the number of vaginal exams, or would you like to be checked at regular intervals?
+ How do you feel about having your water broken to augment labor?
+ Do you want to be offered various positions to push in?
+ Do you want a mirror while pushing?
+ Do you want the option of using a squat bar?

+ Do you want coaching or counting while pushing, or do
  you prefer to push instinctively?

Areas to emphasize that you would like a discussion first:

+ If an episiotomy seems warranted, please gain my
  consent first.
+ Please ask my permission before massaging my
  perineum while pushing.
+ I do/do not want warm compresses applied to my
  perineum during pushing.
+ Please ask before the use of stirrups, unless
  medically necessary.

■ POSTPARTUM

+ Do you want immediate skin-to-skin contact or for
  baby to be cleaned and swaddled first?
+ Do you want delayed cord clamping, if possible?
+ Whom do you want to cut the cord? You? Your partner?
  Big sibling? If anyone specifically does NOT want to
  cut the cord, make a note of that.
+ Do you have plans for banking or donating cord blood?
+ Do you want to take your placenta home?
+ Do you want to see your placenta and learn about it?
+ Do you want visitors in L&D, or do you want them to
  wait until you are moved to your postpartum room?

■ NEWBORN CARE OPTIONS

+ Do you plan to exclusively breastfeed in the hospital, feed baby formula, or a combination?
+ Would you like a lactation consultant to come by on day one or wait until you ask for support?
+ Do you want to delay newborn care procedures like weighing and measuring until after your first experience of bonding and/or breastfeeding?
+ Do you want baby to be given a pacifier?
+ Do you want to delay baby's bath? For how long?
+ Do you want to keep baby with you, or would you like baby to go to the nursery so you can rest?
+ If baby needs to be taken somewhere for a newborn procedure, would you (or your partner) like to go with your baby?
+ Do you plan to circumcise your baby?
+ Do you want erythromycin eye ointment, a vitamin K injection, or the hepatitis B vaccine? You can decline these things but will likely need to sign a waiver. Otherwise, the eye ointment and vitamin K will usually be given toward the end of your baby's first 2 hours of life, and the hepatitis B vaccine within baby's first 12 hours. Emily Oster covers the evidence behind these procedures in her book *Cribsheet* if you're interested in more information.

Chapter 6

The Sixth Month

You're closing in on the third trimester and hopefully still feeling energized. Take this month to check off some practical to-do list items to prepare for baby.

Month 6 Action Plan:

- Find a pediatrician.
- Start working on making room in your home and your budget for baby.
- Get postpartum-ready by stocking up on freezer meals and thinking about how friends and family can support you.

Week 23 Milestones

■ BABY'S STATS

+ Baby is about 11 inches long, weighs 1 pound, and is around the size of a grapefruit.
+ Baby tipped the scales this week! And baby's growth is about to skyrocket, doubling over the next month.

■ MOM'S STATS

Many women experience an increased sex drive this month due to raging hormones and increased blood flow to your sex organs. You may also be loving the way your pregnancy body looks with bigger breasts and a definite baby bump.

■ NOT-TO-MISS APPOINTMENTS

Start interviewing pediatricians. Find out whether they offer things like feeding support (breastfeeding and bottle-feeding), after-hours availability, a 24/7 nurse phone line, and separate waiting rooms for sick and well children. Most importantly, ask yourself whether you feel comfortable with them and whether they align with your parenting philosophies.

WEEK 23 GOALS

Postpartum Prep Find out whether your insurance will cover any postpartum services like a home nurse or postpartum doula who can offer you day or nighttime help.

Make Room As nesting instincts start kicking in, try to tackle some organizational projects to get ready for baby. If it involves a ladder or breathing in any fumes, have your partner or a friend take over.

Rejuvenate Treat yourself to a prenatal massage. When booking the appointment, make sure they have a massage therapist who is trained in prenatal massage and has the proper pillows to keep you comfortable.

KEY ADVICE

Pregnancy cravings are likely in full swing. My craving with my first pregnancy was sushi (don't worry, not raw sushi) followed by a chocolate croissant! If you're craving any nonfood items like dirt, clay, or soap, you could be experiencing a condition called pica, a sign of a nutritional deficiency. Let your care provider know.

Week 24 Milestones

■ BABY'S STATS

+ Baby is about 11.8 inches long, weighs 1.3 pounds, and is around the size of a pomegranate.
+ Baby's heartbeat is now strong enough to hear through a stethoscope.

■ MOM'S STATS

The recommended weight gain at this point is about 10 to 15 pounds total, and about a pound per week from now until birth. Of course, there are many variations of "normal" in this department. If your weight gain is stressing you out, step on the scale backward at your appointments and tell your care provider you'd rather not hear your weight.

■ NOT-TO-MISS APPOINTMENTS

This week, you'll have another prenatal visit. Your doctor or midwife will weigh you, check your blood pressure, have you provide a urine sample, measure your fundal height (length from your pubic bone to the top of your uterus), and listen to baby's heartbeat. You will also be given information about your glucose test, which will occur sometime during the next month.

WEEK 24 GOALS

Postpartum Prep Prepare freezer meals for postpartum. I recommend prepping slow-cooker meals for which you can put all the ingredients into a gallon-sized bag and freeze them. Your third trimester can get really busy, so start checking things like this off your list now.

Budget Boot Camp Look at your monthly income and expenses and then calculate how your income may change during maternity leave. Do you need to cut back on some expenses?

KEY ADVICE

There's a significant increase in vaginal discharge during pregnancy called leukorrhea. The sheer quantity can be a bit alarming. It's typically white and milky and shouldn't smell bad. Use a panty liner—not a tampon—and let your care provider know if it's a color other than white or clear, smells bad, or is causing pain or itchiness.

■ BABY'S STATS

+ Baby is about 13.6 inches long, weighs 1.5 pounds, and is around the size of a head of cauliflower.
+ Baby is working on building their fat stores to keep them warm after birth.

■ MOM'S STATS

Your uterus is now about the size of a volleyball and is putting pressure on your pelvic floor, which could cause hemorrhoids. Witch hazel pads can help soothe them.

■ NOT-TO-MISS APPOINTMENTS

Around this week, you'll have your glucose screening to test for gestational diabetes. You'll be given a very sweet Glucola drink with either 75g or 100g of sugar. One hour after drinking it, you'll have your blood drawn to see how your body is processing it. Ask your care provider about alternatives if you're worried about the taste of the Glucola or object to any of the preservatives, flavorings, or dyes in it.

WEEK 25 GOALS

Decision Time Create a short list of baby names. If you're struggling, try looking at your family tree, watching the credits of TV shows and movies, or using a name generator like the one on nameberry.com.

Stay Strong Ina May Gaskin (referred to as the "mother of midwifery") says if you do 300 squats a day during pregnancy, you'll give birth faster. While this may be a bit extreme, try to get a few sets of squats in each day. Try doing 10 squats every time you go to the bathroom. Fun tip: Many public restrooms have a support bar you can use to steady yourself.

KEY ADVICE

There are a lot of products out there that claim to prevent or treat stretch marks, but stretch marks are genetic and probably can't be prevented. However, they do fade with time. It doesn't hurt to use some coconut oil or vitamin E on any stretch marks that pop up to provide itchiness relief.

Testing for and Treating Gestational Diabetes

Gestational diabetes (GD) is a condition in which a woman develops high blood sugar levels during pregnancy.

You will be given a glucose tolerance test between 24 and 28 weeks of pregnancy, and if your results show elevated blood sugar, you will be diagnosed with gestational diabetes. Your care provider will talk to you about your treatment options. Typically, GD can be managed with diet, especially by lowering carbohydrates, and with exercise. If you have a more severe case, you may need an oral medication or insulin shots. In either case, you may be asked to track your blood sugar levels with a finger-prick blood-glucose monitor. You'll test your blood sugar levels when you wake up and after you eat. Your doctor will advise you on what numbers to look out for.

Potential risks of GD include higher blood pressure, premature birth, and high birth weight, which can lead to complications during

delivery. Baby could also have issues keeping their own blood sugar stable after birth.

The good news is that gestational diabetes usually resolves once your baby is born. You will, however, be at an increased risk for developing type 2 diabetes later in life, so speak with your doctor about future health concerns and potential lifestyle changes.

■ BABY'S STATS

+ Baby is about 14 inches long, weighs 2 pounds, and is around the size of a zucchini.
+ Baby is developing more defined sleep patterns. They may sleep when you're on the move (movement lulls babies to sleep) and be ready to party when you lie down.

■ MOM'S STATS

Your placenta is producing antibodies to build up baby's immune system. You're also producing colostrum (first breast milk), which will provide antibodies to baby after birth. You may experience milk leakage or notice dried, crusty flakes on your nipples. This is a great sign that your body is gearing up for baby.

■ NOT-TO-MISS APPOINTMENTS

Take an infant CPR class. This is a potentially lifesaving skill to have, and infant CPR is administered differently than for a child or adult. You can find a class near you on redcross.org.

WEEK 26 GOALS

Rejuvenate Getting a good night's rest is likely getting harder and harder. Try to rest throughout the day when you can. Even if you don't actually take a nap, lying down with your eyes closed can help with your mood and stress levels.

Postpartum Prep Create a list of action items for your family and friends to help with after baby arrives. Some ideas include dog walking, meal prep, laundry, housecleaning, and grocery shopping. Include detailed instructions on where to find items in your house so they aren't asking you a bunch of questions when you should be resting or bonding with baby.

KEY ADVICE

You may experience congestion and even nosebleeds during pregnancy due to hormonal changes as well as increased blood volume. OTC medications won't help in this instance and might not be safe for baby. Try using a humidifier in your room at night. You can also try putting a bit of peppermint essential oil under your nose to clear your airways. (Check the Resources section on page 171 for a link to my blog on which essential oils are safe to use during pregnancy.)

■ BABY'S STATS

+ Baby is about 14.5 inches long, weighs 2 pounds, and is about the size of a cabbage.
+ Baby's showing brain activity and is even having dreams when they sleep. Baby is also starting to recognize your voice as well as those of family members who are around a lot.

■ MOM'S STATS

+ Your uterus has grown from being the size of a volleyball to being the size of a basketball.
+ As baby gets bigger and is practicing breathing, you may start to notice a rhythmic movement—baby has hiccups.

■ NOT-TO-MISS APPOINTMENTS

Tour your hospital's maternity ward. Even if you're planning an out-of-hospital birth, it's a good idea to be familiar with your nearest hospital, in case of transfer. Suggestions for questions to ask on this tour are on page 83.

WEEK 27 GOALS

Gear Up Thanks to the Affordable Care Act of 2010, all health insurance plans are required to cover the cost of a breast pump (rental or to own). Many services will take care of ordering your breast pump for you at no cost, including aeroflowbreastpumps.com. You fill out a simple form, and they take care of everything else.

Make Room If you haven't gotten on the Marie Kondo band-wagon yet, now's the time. Babies tend to bring a lot more stuff into your life. Try to clear out some of your existing clutter to make room for strollers, bouncers, and countless baby blankets.

KEY ADVICE

Another requirement of the Affordable Care Act is that health insurance plans allow for breastfeeding support. Talk to your doctor about getting a pre-authorization form to see a lactation consultant, and contact your insurance company to find out the details of your breastfeeding benefits.

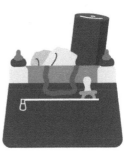

Since many doctors only have privileges at certain hospitals, you may want to look into hospitals early on in your care when choosing a doctor. It's a good idea to ask about the things that are important to you on your hospital tour, because sometimes the official policies differ a bit from day-to-day practice.

Before your tour, search hospital statistics (e.g., cesarean rate) at leapfroggroup.org. Then, on the tour, ask: What is the hospital's cesarean, epidural, episiotomy, and unmedicated birth rate? Even if you found this info on your own, it's good to ask and see whether they are forthcoming or aware.

Search for facilities that have been given the "Baby-Friendly" distinction at babyfriendlyusa.org. The people at improvingbirth.org are also working on creating a "Mother-Friendly" accreditation and search option on their site.

■ POLICIES ON MOBILITY DURING LABOR

+ Do you have wireless monitors or offer intermittent monitoring?
+ Will I have access to a shower or bath? Do you have waterproof monitors?
+ What equipment do you have available, or can I bring my own? (e.g., squat bar, birth ball, peanut ball, birth stool)
+ Do you have volunteer or hospital-staffed doulas available?

■ PAIN RELIEF

Is there a dedicated anesthesia team for L&D? How long does it typically take them to respond once I request pain medication?

■ CESAREAN POLICIES

+ What is the hospital's cesarean rate? (You can check leapfroggroup.org, but it's good to ask and see whether they are forthcoming or aware.)
+ Do you offer routine skin-to-skin contact in the OR?
+ Are doulas welcomed in the OR? What about birth photographers?
+ How many support people are allowed in recovery?

■ NEWBORN CARE

+ Do you encourage baby rooming in with mom?
+ Do you offer routine, uninterrupted, skin-to-skin contact for an hour after birth?
+ What are your breastfeeding rates? What kind of lactation support is available?

■ NICU

+ What are the procedures and routines for a premature infant or a baby who has special needs at birth?
+ What level NICU do you have? If they have a lower-level NICU, ask what the transfer hospital would be.
+ What are the visitation rules for the NICU?
+ Will our pediatrician have rights at the hospital/NICU?
+ Is skin-to-skin contact/kangaroo care with baby supported? How frequently?
+ Does the NICU have a dedicated lactation consultant? Are breast pumps available to use in the NICU?

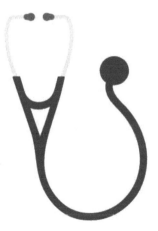

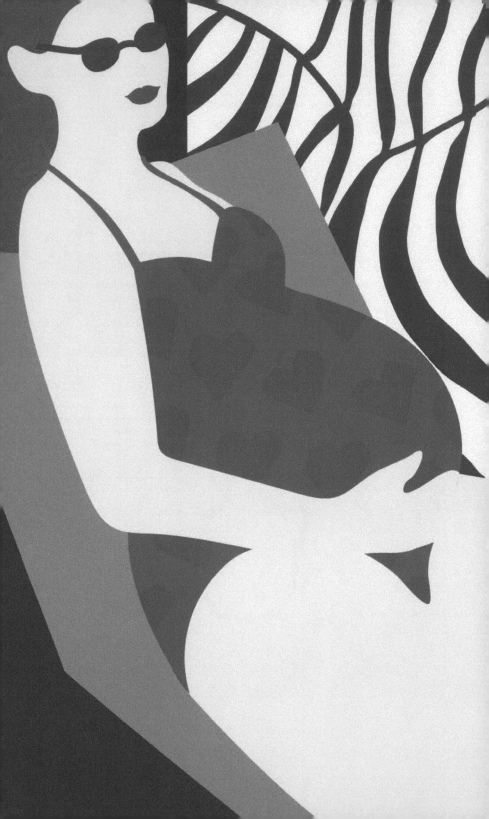

PART III

The Third Trimester

You've made it to the third and final trimester of pregnancy. And you're likely starting to feel pretty stretched—both physically, as your baby continues to grow, and emotionally, as you start to imagine life with a baby in it. Excited and anxious to meet your baby? Great! But it's also normal to be nervous about what childbirth and postpartum will bring.

Now, your prenatal appointments will increase from once a month to every two weeks, then once a week. You'll be tested for group B strep, and baby's growth and position will be monitored and could affect where or how you give birth. This is the time to start thinking more about your birth preferences and preparing for healing postpartum.

Input from family, friends, and total strangers will likely increase as everyone wants to know whether you're getting an epidural, whether you're sure it's not twins, and are you really *still* pregnant? Ignore the negative, embrace the positive, and continue to be gentle with yourself. Find rest whenever possible, and spend time with your partner or friends and family doing the things you love most. This is your time to focus on growing a human and preparing to mother your baby. It's hard work.

In this section, you'll find information and goals to focus on during these last months of pregnancy. As your belly grows, you might feel like you're going to be pregnant forever, or it may dawn on you one day out of the blue that your baby will be here in a matter of weeks! As your estimated due date approaches, we'll focus on getting you ready for birth and the tender weeks that follow.

Chapter 7

The Seventh Month

You'll likely start to see your doctor or midwife every two weeks instead of every four. They will be checking on your vitals, keeping an eye out for things like preeclampsia, and also checking on baby's growth.

Month 7 Action Plan:

- Pay attention to baby's movements, thinking about patterns and frequency, so you can be aware of any changes.

- Think about your preferences for childbirth.

- Begin preparing for postpartum by talking to any friends or family who may be coming to support you once baby arrives, as well as your postpartum doula if you've hired one.

Week 28 Milestones

■ BABY'S STATS

+ Baby is about 15 inches long, weighs 2.2 pounds, and is around the size of a head of lettuce.
+ Many babies will turn head down at this point, but 25 percent of babies are breech (bottom down) before 28 weeks. That number drops to 7 percent by 32 weeks.

■ MOM'S STATS

Many women experience heaviness or soreness in their pelvic floor muscles during the third trimester. Consider getting a maternity support belt, especially if you are on your feet a lot or have any travel plans coming up.

■ NOT-TO-MISS APPOINTMENTS

You'll have a routine prenatal checkup this week. Your care provider will weigh you, check your blood pressure, and test your urine for elevated protein and sugar levels.

They'll also measure your belly to ensure baby's growing on track, listen to baby's heart rate, and ask about baby's movements.

WEEK 28 GOALS

Stay Strong At your appointment this week, most care providers will ask you to start keeping track of baby's movements. There's a handy app called Count the Kicks that can help you remember to do this.

Budget Boot Camp Consider adding a 529 college-savings plan to your baby registry. This is a tax-advantaged way to save for baby's college. It's a long way off, but if you start saving now, your money earns interest over the next 18 years. Check out collegebacker.com, a free service that will help you set the fund up even before baby is born.

KEY ADVICE

According to the American Congress of Obstetricians and Gynecologists (ACOG), between 14 and 23 percent of women will experience some symptoms of depression and anxiety during pregnancy. If you're one of them, please do not deal with this alone. Talk to your care provider and consider seeing a mental health practitioner. More information on perinatal mood disorders is on page 100.

Week 29 Milestones

■ BABY'S STATS

+ Baby is about 15.5 inches long, weighs 2.75 pounds, and is about the size of an acorn squash.
+ Baby's eyes are no longer fused shut, and baby is practicing blinking.

■ MOM'S STATS

Many women experience carpal tunnel syndrome (tingling and numbness in the hands) during the third trimester. It can be worse at night, especially if you've been using your hands all day at work. Try soaking in a tub or icing your hands, and know that it should subside after pregnancy.

■ NOT-TO-MISS APPOINTMENTS

If you're experiencing urinary leaking when you sneeze or exercise, consider seeing a pelvic floor physical therapist. They can give you exercises to strengthen your pelvic floor and help alleviate some of those symptoms. You don't have to wait until baby arrives to get started.

WEEK 29 GOALS

Birth Day Listen to birth stories. My podcast, *The Birth Hour*, has hundreds of all types, and many listeners report that hearing other women's stories was their greatest preparation for childbirth. You can listen for free in any podcast app or at thebirthhour.com.

Symptoms 101 If you're feeling forgetful or foggy-minded, know that "pregnancy brain" is a real thing. Aside from poor sleep, mental fogginess could be related to a decrease in brain cell volume during the third trimester. The research isn't completely settled on this symptom, but anecdotally, I can tell you most women I know experience some form of this during pregnancy and after they give birth, too.

KEY ADVICE

During pregnancy, many women experience increased levels of anxiety. Pay attention to what is causing you stress, and try to cut it out until after baby is born. For example, I tried to watch A Handmaid's Tale *while I was pregnant with my third baby, and I would feel the anxiety creeping up from my stomach to my chest. I stopped watching and immediately felt relief.*

Week 30 Milestones

■ BABY'S STATS

+ Baby is about 16 inches long, weighs 3 pounds, and is around the size of a large cabbage.
+ Baby is now able to grasp their foot, an adorable skill they will use once they are born to grasp your finger.

■ MOM'S STATS

You may be experiencing overheating as your metabolism increases and your belly continues to grow. This can be especially uncomfortable in hot or humid climates. Be sure to drink lots of water, and go for a swim if you can. Another great trick is a drop of peppermint essential oil behind your ears. (Check the Resources section on page 171 for a link to my blog on which essential oils are safe to use during pregnancy.)

■ NOT-TO-MISS APPOINTMENTS

If you booked those maternity photos we talked about earlier, your photo shoot is likely here. Looking for a budget-friendly option? Many photographers offer mini sessions, where they batch a few shoots in a row on a specific day.

WEEK 30 GOALS

Make Room Clear your schedule as much as possible for the first 12 weeks after baby is born. I recommend Heng Ou's book *The First Forty Days: The Essential Art of Nourishing the New Mother*. It covers information on healing foods and practices for recovering from childbirth as you step into your role as a mother.

Birth Day Start researching pain-relief options during childbirth. If you're having an out-of-hospital birth, your options will be referred to as coping strategies and can include movement, massage, counter pressure, and water. If you're giving birth at a hospital, you'll have the additional options of IV meds, an epidural, and possibly nitrous oxide.

KEY ADVICE

Be aware of informed consent in your maternity care. Informed consent means your care provider should never be doing anything to you, or your baby, without first explaining it to you, answering your questions, and waiting for your consent. I highly recommend the book **Birth without Fear** *by January Harshe for more on being an informed consumer of maternity care and feeling empowered in your decision-making.*

■ BABY'S STATS

+ Baby is about 16.2 inches long, weighs about 3.3 pounds, and is around the size of a coconut.
+ Baby's brain is forming wrinkles so it can store more brain cells.

■ MOM'S STATS

Braxton-Hicks contractions might be picking up at this stage and may cause you to wonder whether you're experiencing preterm labor. Unlike the real thing, Braxton-Hicks contractions shouldn't be painful or come in a pattern.

■ NOT-TO-MISS APPOINTMENTS

This is a great time to have your baby shower, if you decided to have one. Consider having it at someone else's home so you aren't worrying about getting things party-ready or dealing with cleanup. You shouldn't feel beholden to any traditional ideas of what a baby shower should be. Maybe you'd rather just go out to lunch with a few friends or have a couple's shower so all of the attention isn't only on you!

WEEK 31 GOALS

Birth Day If you're having a hospital birth, make sure you're preregistered. You'll still sign paperwork when you check in, but this can save you from spelling out your street name between contractions. You may be able to take care of it on your hospital tour or complete it online or by mail.

Postpartum Prep Attend a La Leche League or other lactation group meeting. You can find one at llli.org. I made some mom friends before my first baby was even born through La Leche League. If you're not interested in learning about breast-feeding, you could connect with moms at prenatal exercise or yoga classes, childbirth classes, or online groups.

KEY ADVICE

If you're having a boy, you'll have a big decision to make right away—whether to circumcise or not. Circumcision is a surgical procedure to remove the tip of your baby's foreskin. In the United States, about 50 percent of baby boys are circumcised. These numbers are from 2009, and trends showed then that rates were declining. Childbirth educator Stephanie Spitzer-Hanks wrote an article for The Birth Hour *on the evidence around circumcision, which you can read at thebirthhour.com.*

Chapter 8

The Eighth Month

Baby is starting to take up more room and may be getting into position for birth. If you're planning to take a childbirth class, this is a good time to do so.

Month 8 Action Plan:

- Learn about the symptoms of perinatal mood disorders and have a plan in place if you experience any of them.
- Start gathering supplies for your birth and educate yourself on the process of labor.
- Learn about baby's position and how it may affect labor.

Perinatal Mood and Anxiety Disorders (PMADs)

About 15 to 20 percent of new mothers experience postpartum depression (PPD), characterized by extreme sadness or loss of interest in your baby, and about 10 percent of new mothers experience postpartum anxiety (PPA), which is constant worry and a loss of balance or control. The main cause is hormonal shifts coupled with any or all of the following: lack of sleep, poor nutrition, a high-needs baby, health issues for mom or baby, isolation, or inadequate support from your partner or family. PPA can be experienced on its own or in conjunction with PPD.

Since many of the causes are situational, not just hormonal, about 25 percent of partners experience depression and/or anxiety after baby arrives, as well.

Symptoms to watch for include:

- ✦ Feeling sad or depressed
- ✦ Feeling irritable, angry, or even enraged
- ✦ Being unable to bond with baby
- ✦ Having difficulty eating or drinking
- ✦ Feeling panicky or anxious

- Experiencing disturbing thoughts that you can't get out of your head
- Feeling like you're "going crazy" or are "out of control"
- Feeling like you should have never become a mom
- Being concerned that you might hurt yourself or your baby

You and your partner, or support people, should be educated on these symptoms prior to childbirth. If you do experience any of these symptoms, and they are persistent or last beyond two weeks postpartum, please seek help. Your care provider should be knowledgeable in treating postpartum mood disorders, but if you are not feeling understood and supported, find a different provider. Listen to your gut, and if you think you need help, don't wait.

Postpartumprogress.com has 24/7 phone and text support helplines for English- and Spanish-speaking mothers, and the helpline staff are educated in less common postpartum disorders, like postpartum obsessive-compulsive disorder and postpartum post-traumatic stress disorder.

These are treatable illnesses. Whether you need medication, therapy, supplements, or a support group, there are options for you. You have to prioritize taking care of yourself so you can take care of your baby.

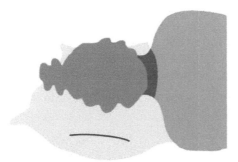

Week 32 Milestones

■ BABY'S STATS

+ Baby is about 16 to 17 inches long, weighs 3.5 to 4 pounds, and is around the size of a cantaloupe.
+ Baby's eyes are developing rapidly. They can now focus on large close-up objects as well as adjust to darkness.

■ MOM'S STATS

At this point in pregnancy, you're gaining about a pound each week, and about half of that is going toward increasing baby's weight.

■ NOT-TO-MISS APPOINTMENTS

Seeing a chiropractor can help alleviate back pain during late pregnancy. And chiropractors who specialize in seeing pregnant women can adjust your pelvis and help baby get into the best position for birth. Look for a chiropractor who is Webster certified. A good place to start is icpa4kids.com.

WEEK 32 GOALS

Gear Up If you're planning a home birth, your midwife will give you a list of items you need to have on hand, including a birth kit that has things like an umbilical cord clamp. Go ahead and order those now so they arrive by week 36.

Make Room Focus on making your bedroom the coziest place in the house. It should spark some serious joy, because you're about to be spending a lot of time there. Many women focus on preparing the nursery, which is super fun, but baby will likely be rooming-in with you for at least a few weeks if not months.

Around 7 percent of babies are still breech (head up) at this point, but only about 3 percent are still breech at full term.

In 2001, a study came out recommending cesarean sections for all breech babies. It was later debunked, but practices had already begun to shift in the direction of surgical birth for breech babies. I recommend birthinginstincts.com and the film Heads Up: The Disappearing Art of Vaginal Breech Delivery *for more information. Spinningbabies.com is a great resource on baby's positioning, as well.*

Week 33 Milestones

■ BABY'S STATS

+ Baby is about 17.2 inches long, weighs approximately 4.3 pounds, and is around the size of a pineapple.

+ Baby swallows up to a pint of amniotic fluid each day and is learning how to coordinate sucking and swallowing while breathing.

■ MOM'S STATS

You may experience shortness of breath, especially if you're exerting yourself, and by exerting yourself, I mean walking up a couple of stairs. Try slowing down and decreasing your activity level. It can also be helpful to stand up straight with your shoulders back to give your lungs more room to expand in your increasingly cramped chest.

■ NOT-TO-MISS APPOINTMENTS

Certain indicators mean you could face additional challenges with breastfeeding, including having flat or inverted nipples, or if your breasts haven't changed in size or density during pregnancy. Ask your doctor or midwife for a referral to a lactation consultant prior to baby's arrival, or find a lactation consultant near you using the directories at ilca.org or uslca.org.

WEEK 33 GOALS

Postpartum Prep Make padsicles. Yes, you read that right. Padsicles can be extremely soothing to your perineum after giving birth, but making them takes a little time, so I recommend tackling this before baby arrives. You'll need maxi pads, witch hazel, aloe vera gel, and plastic wrap. You can also add essential oils like lavender and helichrysum.*

1. Unfold the pad, but don't remove it from the outer plastic wrap.
2. Apply aloe vera gel liberally.
3. Apply witch hazel sparingly (you don't want to use up all the absorbency of the pad).
4. Add a couple of drops of essential oils.*
5. Refold and wrap in plastic wrap.
6. Place in freezer.

*Check the Resources section on page 171 for a link to my blog on which essential oils are safe to use during pregnancy.

KEY ADVICE

Gathering supplies for your postpartum recovery is one of the best things you can do to make those first few weeks go more smoothly. You'll particularly want supplies to help with your healing and to aid in breast-feeding, if you plan to breastfeed. There's a list of my favorite items for postpartum moms on page 129.

Week 34 Milestones

■ BABY'S STATS

+ Baby is about 17.7 inches long, weighs about 4.75 pounds, and is around the size of a butternut squash.

+ Baby is now able to see color, although the only color available is the red inside of your uterus.

■ MOM'S STATS

As baby starts to take up more room, there is less amniotic fluid to cushion baby's movements. As a result, you may start to feel more sharp jabs and kicks. You can even watch your belly protrude when baby extends an arm or leg.

■ NOT-TO-MISS APPOINTMENTS

If you and your doctor have decided on a planned cesarean birth, you'll likely be scheduling baby's birthday at your next appointment, usually for around 39 to 40 weeks. With a planned cesarean (versus an unplanned one), you can voice your preferences in advance. Research "family-centered" or "gentle" cesarean births and discuss them with your doctor.

WEEK 34 GOALS

Birth Day Save these phone numbers in your phone (if they apply to you):

+ Your care provider and birth location
+ Doula or other support person
+ Birth photographer
+ Sitter for any pets or older children

- *In addition to plugging the numbers into your phone, write out a list and put it on your refrigerator so it's in plain sight.*

Gear Up If you have any formal occasions in these last few weeks, you'll likely need a maternity dress—and fancy maternity dresses can be hard to come by. I recommend checking out Rent the Runway's maternity section.

KEY ADVICE

The World Health Organization has determined that the rate for medically necessary cesarean sections should be around 10 to 15 percent. The United States has a rate of over 30 percent. This data illustrates that many cesarean sections in the United States are not medically necessary. Look at evidencebasedbirth.com and research the evidence.

Week 35 Milestones

■ BABY'S STATS

+ Baby is about 18 inches long, weighs about 5 pounds, and is around the size of a spaghetti squash.
+ Baby is mostly working on fattening up at this point. Babies build up what's called brown fat, which functions to keep them warm once they are born.

■ MOM'S STATS

You may start to notice swollen ankles and feet, especially if you live in a hot climate. This is usually a normal pregnancy symptom, but if it's severe or accompanied by swelling in other areas, remember that it could be a sign of preeclampsia, and contact your care provider right away.

■ NOT-TO-MISS APPOINTMENTS

Group B strep tests are typically given between 35 and 37 weeks. Group B streptococcus (GBS) is a bacteria that lives in the intestines and urinary tract. If you are GBS positive, you'll be offered antibiotics during labor through either an IV or an injection. As with any prenatal test, you do have a choice and can discuss your options with your care provider.

WEEK 35 GOALS

Birth Day Call your doctor or midwife if your water breaks, you have any bleeding, you are feeling painful or menstrual-like contractions, or your contractions are coming in a regular pattern and the intervals are getting closer together.

Postpartum Prep Do you have pets? If so, now is a good time to start planning for who will take care of them. Regardless of whether you're having a hospital birth, birth-center birth, or home birth, labor and bonding with baby will take all your attention.

You will hear mixed responses from birth profession-als when it comes to writing a birth plan. In The Birth Hour's childbirth course, we refer to creating a list of "birth preferences," because the fact of the matter is that birth is unpredictable. Suggestions of things to consider when writing out your birth preferences are on page 67.

Feeding Your Baby

In the United States, about 82 percent of mothers breastfeed their babies at birth. That number drops to 52 percent by the time baby is 6 months old. Feeding your baby is often one of the more emotionally and physically difficult things you will do as a new mother. Whether by breast or by bottle, you'll be feeding your newborn at least every two to three hours for the first few weeks.

If you plan to breastfeed, I encourage you to seek support both during pregnancy and after baby arrives. Yes, breastfeeding *is* natural, but it doesn't always *come* naturally. You may face physical issues like cracked nipples, inverted or flat nipples, or latch problems. Or your baby may not be gaining weight as quickly as your pediatrician would like. Or maybe baby is gassy due to oversupply and a strong letdown.

All this is to say: Feeding your baby is complicated, and you should be supported whatever your choice.

Reach out for help when needed, listen to your gut, and know that whatever you decide, you are feeding your baby with love. If you're interested in looking closely at the data on the short- and long-term benefits of breastfeeding, I recommend Emily Oster's book *Cribsheet*.

Feeding Supplies

This list is focused on items to help you with feeding your baby, but keep in mind that you're going to need to eat, too! Have a snack station near your bed or favorite chair full of high-protein items like trail mix, protein bars, and lactation cookies—a great excuse to eat a cookie any time of day. I also recommend a large cup with a straw. I was so thirsty while breastfeeding that I had two 30-ounce cups near me at all times!

■ BOTTLE-FEEDING

+ Bottles and bottle brushes

If pumping:

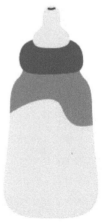

+ Breast pump (get one for free through insurance using a site like aeroflowbreastpumps.com)
+ Hands-free pumping bra, or simply cut two holes in a sports bra
+ Milk storage bags or Milkies milk tray
+ Coconut oil or nipple balm to lubricate your pump flanges before pumping

If formula feeding:

+ Formula (find more info on page 149)
+ Filtered water if using powdered formula. You can pre-make a pitcher full of formula each day to save time. Just remember you need to use it within 24 hours.

■ BREASTFEEDING

+ Breastfeeding pillow – My Brest Friend offers great support, especially for cesarean recovery.
+ Breast pads – disposable and cloth
+ Milk catcher like the Milkies Milk Saver or Haakaa
+ Stretchy nursing tank and comfy nursing sleep bra – Again, I love Kindred Bravely, especially if you are larger-chested, as they have "busty" sizing.
+ Nipple care – gel packs, nipple butter, lanolin, and Amorini Silver Nipple Soothers
+ Nipple shells – Different from nipple shields, these allow your nipples to air out without rubbing against your clothes.

Chapter 9

The Ninth Month

The final month of pregnancy! Can you believe it? Of course, it could still be another six weeks, as babies are not considered post-term until after 42 weeks. I always recommend planning on baby being "late," so you aren't too disappointed. On the other hand, baby could be born tomorrow, which is definitely exciting!

Month 9 Action Plan:

- Make sure you're ready to transport baby with a properly installed car seat.

- Finish putting together everything you need to bring with you to the hospital or birth center. See Hospital Bag Packing Suggestions on page 120. If you're having a home birth, make sure your supplies are accessible and labeled if needed.

Week 36 Milestones

■ BABY'S STATS

+ Baby is about 18.5 inches long, weighs 6 pounds, and is around the size of a papaya.
+ Baby's lungs are maturing and producing surfactant, a substance that will help baby's lungs take in air outside your womb.

■ MOM'S STATS

You may notice a difference in the way baby's movements feel. As baby starts to run out of room, you'll feel fewer kicks and jabs and more rolls and shifting.

■ NOT-TO-MISS APPOINTMENTS

Starting this week, you will have prenatal checkups every week until baby arrives. If you have any outstanding questions about labor and delivery, now is the time to ask.

WEEK 36 GOALS

Decision Time Write out a birth announcement ahead of time with a list of email addresses or phone numbers for your partner or a friend to send it on your behalf. If you have any strained relationships, have someone else share the news for you, so you aren't putting any unnecessary stress on yourself right after giving birth.

Gear Up Get your infant car seat installed and have it checked by a certified child passenger safety technician (CPST). According to the *Journal of Pediatrics*, 95 percent of infant car seats have at least one installation error. You can find a local CPST at safekids.org or thetotsquad.com.

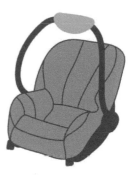

KEY ADVICE

The first hour or so after baby is born is referred to as the "golden hour," and it's a wonderful time for skin-to-skin bonding with your baby. Skin-to-skin contact is proven to help baby regulate their heart rate, blood pressure, and temperature. If you're feeling shaky, nauseous, or overwhelmed, it's okay to hand baby off for a bit. Do what feels right to you.

■ BABY'S STATS

+ Baby is about 19 inches long, weighs 6.5 pounds, and is around the size of a head of romaine lettuce.
+ Baby is now considered term and is ready for life on the outside. Over the next few weeks baby's lungs will continue to mature, and baby will keep gaining weight—about half a pound a week.

■ MOM'S STATS

You may be experiencing fatigue as you carry an extra 30 pounds around in your abdomen. Plus, sleep can be difficult toward the end of pregnancy. Rest up if you can, and if you are one of those women who feels great right up until baby's arrival—enjoy!

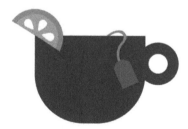

■ NOT-TO-MISS APPOINTMENTS

If it's important to you, get your hair cut. A low-maintenance hairstyle will make postpartum much easier when you suddenly don't have time for your daily styling routine. If you get your hair colored, consider balayage instead of traditional highlights or all-over color, because it grows out much more gradually and will need less maintenance.

WEEK 37 GOALS

Career Coach Finalize your maternity leave plans. If you work for a company, schedule a meeting with your team and discuss how your work will be handled in your absence. If you work for yourself, try to frontload your work so you can unplug for at least a few weeks. Set an out-of-office response in your email that is ready for you to activate when the time comes.

Gear Up Sterilize your breast pump parts and read over the manual. When you've never used one before, breast pumps can be a little intimidating. Better to learn now, before there is a baby in the mix.

Week 38 Milestones

■ BABY'S STATS

+ Baby is about 19 to 20 inches long, weighs approx- imately 6.75 pounds, and is around the size of a mini watermelon.
+ Baby is practicing for birth by turning from side to side, breathing in amniotic fluid, and sucking their thumb.

■ MOM'S STATS

You may be able to breathe a little easier in the last few weeks of pregnancy as baby "drops" into your pelvis, creating more space for your lungs. Also referred to as "lightening," this is something that first-time moms almost always experience from two to four weeks before delivery. For subsequent pregnancies, baby may not drop until labor begins.

■ NOT-TO-MISS APPOINTMENTS

You'll continue to see your doctor or midwife each week up until 40 weeks. If you go past 40 weeks, you may start to have twice-a-week appointments. At your appoint- ments, some care providers will offer to do a cervical check, so they can tell whether your cervix is thinning (effacement) or opening (dilation).

WEEK 38 GOALS

Gear Up Wash all of baby's newborn clothes and blankets using a nontoxic detergent—¼ cup of baking soda works well, too. Folding tiny, adorable clothes is a fun way to pass the time as you wait for baby to arrive. Try to get caught up on your own laundry, as well, because it will all start to multiply postpartum.

Make Room Put a waterproof sheet under your fitted sheet in case your water breaks in bed. This is also a necessity for home births and can come in handy for anyone postpartum when you'll have postpartum bleeding and leaking breast milk, and will be holding a baby who could spit up or pee in the middle of a diaper change.

KEY ADVICE

There is little evidence that cervical changes indicate when you will go into labor, or even how long labor will last. It is always your right to decline having cervical checks prior to or even during labor. Remember: informed consent! Many women find hearing those numbers discouraging when they think they should be more dilated than they are at any given time. Keep in mind that many women will dilate quickly once labor starts, while for others it's a slow and steady process. When it comes to childbirth, there are many variations of normal.

Hospital Bag Packing Suggestions

This is a pretty comprehensive list, so feel free to take or leave whatever makes sense for you and the birth you're planning. Many doulas will bring some of these things for you, and some hospitals will have some of this stuff on hand.

■ LABOR & DELIVERY

+ Photo ID and insurance card
+ Copies of your birth preferences, aka "birth plan"
+ Birth ball and peanut ball
+ Heating pad
+ Snacks
+ What will help relax you? Consider birth affirmations, music, essential oils, twinkle lights/fake candles, a fan, or massage oil. (Check the Resources section on page 171 for a link to my blog on which essential oils are safe to use during pregnancy.)

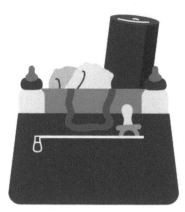

■ POSTPARTUM

+ Peppermint essential oil. Put a couple of drops in the toilet, and the vapor from the oil will encourage your first postpartum pee when it reaches the perineum.
+ Earth Mama Organics perineal spray and balm
+ Stool softener
+ Cesarean support panties
+ Ice chest if you're planning to bring home your placenta

■ BREASTFEEDING

+ Nipple balm
+ Reusable breast pads
+ Nursing pillow
+ Milkies Milk Saver or Haakaa

■ CLOTHES & ACCESSORIES

+ Birth gown (if you want an option other than the hospital gown)
+ Robe
+ Shower shoes and slippers
+ Hair ties
+ Sleep/nursing bra
+ Sweaters for you and your partner (hospital rooms can get quite chilly)
+ Comfy change of clothes for you and your partner
+ Eye mask and earplugs
+ Extra-long phone charger

■ TOILETRIES

+ Lip balm
+ Face wash and lotion
+ Toothbrush and toothpaste
+ Toiletries for your partner
+ Nice to have: dry shampoo, makeup, and makeup remover wipes

■ FOR BABY

+ Wipes for sensitive skin
+ Pacifier (if you want baby to have one other than what the hospital provides)
+ Blankets and coming-home outfit
+ Properly installed car seat

You can find more info at thebirthhour.com. If you're planning a home birth, many of these things will be on hand, but it doesn't hurt to go over the list and organize what you think you might need. Your midwife will also likely have you order a birth kit with additional supplies.

Week 39 Milestones

■ BABY'S STATS

+ Baby is 19 to 21 inches long, weighs 7 to 8 pounds, and is about the size of a honeydew melon.
+ Baby's skull remains soft so it can squeeze through the birth canal. You may notice a cone shape to baby's head at birth, but it usually rounds out within a day or two.

■ MOM'S STATS

Once baby drops into your pelvis, you may trade short-ness of breath for something many moms refer to as "lightning crotch." This is a sharp or shooting pain in your vagina or rectum caused by pressure from baby on your nerve endings. It can stop you in your tracks.

■ NOT-TO-MISS APPOINTMENTS

If you're having a planned cesarean birth, your doctor may recommend you speak with the anesthesiologist about any prior medical conditions or reactions to drugs that could cause complications. The anesthesiologist is often the one making the call on who gets to be in the room during surgery, so even if your doctor said it was fine to have your partner and doula, it's a good idea to check with the anesthesiologist, as well.

WEEK 39 GOALS

Make Room Treat yourself to a housecleaning service or ask for it as a gift from a family member who is wondering how they can help you. Having a clean home—that you didn't have to clean yourself—will take off some stress as you lead up to your due date.

Gear Up Studies have shown that having baby in your room with you for at least six months reduces the risk of SIDS (sudden infant death syndrome). The American Academy of Pediatrics recommends babies sleep in their parent's room, but in their own bassinet or co-sleeper with nothing else in it.

Waiting to cut baby's umbilical cord (delayed cord clamping) even as little as 30 seconds can increase your baby's blood volume by as much as one third. This in turn increases your baby's iron stores, which are crucial for brain development. If you're having a cesarean birth, your doctor probably won't want to wait minutes, but as long as the baby is breathing well at birth, even a few seconds is better than immediate clamping.

Week 40 Milestones

■ BABY'S STATS

+ Baby is 19 to 21 inches long, weighs between 7 and 10 pounds, and is about the size of a watermelon.
+ Baby has shed most of their vernix (the waxy coating on their skin), so sometimes later-term babies have some dry skin when they are born.

■ MOM'S STATS

You might be feeling ready but nervous at the same time. Your body is likely doing the work of preparing for labor without you even noticing. Braxton-Hicks contractions might be increasing, and your cervix may be dilating and thinning.

■ NOT-TO-MISS APPOINTMENTS

Going past your due date can be emotionally difficult. I recommend having something fun planned for this day that you can look forward to. It won't completely take your mind off the fact that you're still pregnant, but it will give you something else to look forward to if you wake up and haven't gone into labor.

WEEK 40 GOALS

Rejuvenate Get a pedicure. Even if you're not someone who normally gets pedicures, this is your time. You can't reach your feet easily, and you probably won't be heading to the nail salon anytime soon with a newborn. So enjoy having your legs massaged, and choose a fun nail color that makes you smile.

Symptoms 101 You may notice an increase in cervical mucus and can even have a large glob come out that may have a pink or brown tinge to it. This is your mucus plug or "bloody show." Despite sounding like a horror movie, it's completely normal and could be a positive sign that labor will begin soon.

At 40 weeks, many care providers will start to talk about induction possibilities. As with most things surrounding birth, there are pros and cons to induction. Talk to your care provider about your concerns and preferences. It can be a hard decision, and it's something we spend a lot of time educating on in **The Birth Hour's** *childbirth course.*

Week 40 to 42 Milestones

■ BABY'S STATS

+ Baby is 21 to 22 inches long, weighs around 7 to 10 pounds, and is about the size of a newborn baby!
+ Your baby can recognize the sound of your voice. Many babies will be crying when they're born, and once they hear Mom's voice, they stop and look up at her. It's pretty amazing!

■ MOM'S STATS

I know how hard it is to still be pregnant, but you aren't alone. About 30 percent of pregnancies go past the estimated due date. My first baby was born 16 days after her estimated due date, and my second was 13 days after.

Remember it's an *estimated* due date, and many factors can play into it being a bit off.

■ NOT-TO-MISS APPOINTMENTS

Typically, when you go past your due date, your doctor or midwife will order a biophysical profile and/or a non-stress test. The biophysical profile is an ultrasound to look at baby's movement, tone, heart rate, and breathing, plus check on the level of amniotic fluid. In the non-stress test, you'll be hooked up to a fetal monitor and push a button when you feel movement. Your care provider will look to see how baby's heart rate responds to its movements.

WEEK 40 TO 42 GOALS

This Is Love I know you are probably Googling all the ways to start labor, and "have sex" is coming up over and over again. Having an orgasm causes uterine contractions and could help start labor. If you're not feeling up for sex, just know that it probably won't start labor unless your body is ready.

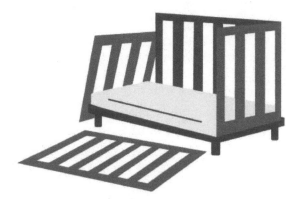

Make Room For many women, starting a project can be just the thing to get their body ready for labor. Maybe it's that you're taking your mind off still being pregnant, or maybe your baby is already eager to interrupt you, but it can't hurt to try!

Postpartum Plan and Recovery Supply List

Write or type up a postpartum plan for who your support people are going to be. Below are some suggestions of people to have on hand to create your own makeshift "village." Speak with them ahead of time and let them know you are planning to reach out when you need their help. Your loved ones *want* to help and will be honored that you trust them with this responsibility. Write down names and numbers of family, friends, and professionals whom you can call when you need help during the day, evening, or even overnight.

+ Include people you can call for emotional support and a little empathy when you need to vent. Having a therapist lined up is never a bad idea, even if you don't end up needing one.
+ Whom will you call when you run into challenges with breastfeeding? Friends who are knowledgeable, lactation consultants, and support groups are all great options.
+ Who is willing to help with your pets and/or older children?
+ Who has offered to bring meals? Have a friend create a meal calendar for you at mealtrain.com, and make a plan for how many nights a week you'll order takeout.
+ Write down names of friends, relatives, or a professional cleaning service you can call when housework feels overwhelming.

As far as what you'll need, a lot of it will depend on how your birth goes and whether you run into any breastfeeding issues, but this is a good starting point. You can always keep the receipts and wait to open things until you need them. That being said, I definitely recommend spending more time thinking about what *you* will need postpartum than what the baby will need. Babies don't need much in the first few weeks!

■ BATHROOM NEEDS

+ Peri bottle or bidet – Many women swear by the FridaBaby MomWasher, and I personally am obsessed with the Tushy, which is an affordable bidet that easily attaches to your toilet.
+ Squatty Potty – This is a stool for your feet that can be helpful postpartum. Your first poop after giving birth can be, um, difficult. This can help relieve some of the pressure on your perineum.
+ Stool softener like Colace
+ Flushable wipes

■ PERINEUM AND HEMORRHOIDS

+ Witch hazel pads for hemorrhoids and stitches
+ Dermoplast or other lidocaine spray and Preparation H cream for hemorrhoids
+ Earth Mama Organics Perineal Spray and Perineal Balm
+ Padsicles (recipe on page 104), cold packs from the hospital (also available on Amazon), or Rachel's Remedy Down There Relief Pack
+ Birthsong Botanicals Postpartum Herb Bath or Earth Mama Organics Herbal Sitz Bath
+ Sitz bath or a clean bathtub to use with postpartum herb bath

+ Inflatable donut cushion to sit on, or use the Boppy breastfeeding pillow .
+ Comfy underwear. I love the postpartum underwear from Kindred Bravely. They are high-waisted, so if you had a cesarean, they won't rub your scar.

POSTPARTUM BLEEDING

+ Heating pad and AfterEase tincture for postpartum cramping
+ Adult diapers like Depends
+ Large maxi pads and mesh boyshort underwear (available from the hospital or on Amazon)
+ Reusable "mama cloth" pads. Normal duration for postpartum bleeding is anywhere from two to eight weeks. You shouldn't use a menstrual cup or tampons for postpartum bleeding.
+ Waterproof sheet or bed pads to protect your mattress

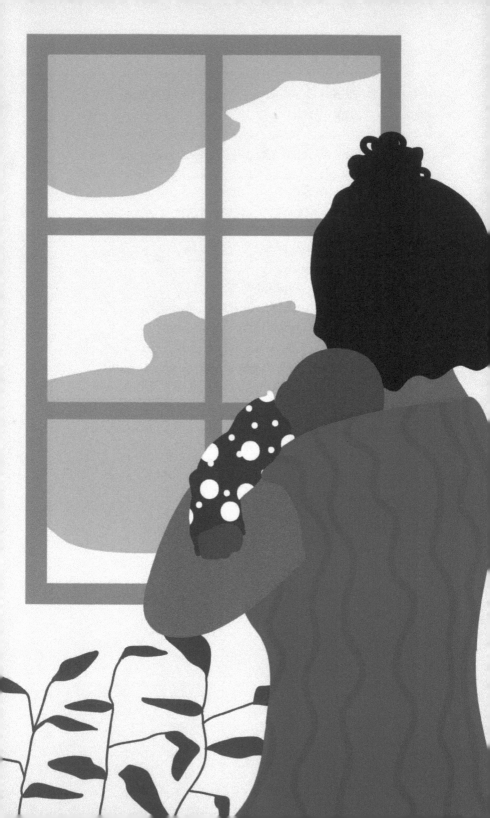

PART IV

The "Fourth Trimester"

Congratulations are in order—you did it! I truly wish I could reach out through this book and give you the biggest hug ever! If I think hard enough back on my own postpartum experiences, I start welling up with emotion. It's such a raw, tender, beautiful, and unbelievably challenging time. Your baby is here, and life is about to become one big blur for a few months.

The first 12 weeks of your baby's life are referred to as the *fourth trimester*. Baby is transitioning from the womb to the outside world but is completely helpless in comparison to other mammals at birth. They will rely on you for absolutely everything.

This is also a huge transformation for you as a woman. Anthropologists refer to the process of becoming a mother as "matrescence." Similar to adolescence, this is a massive transition hormonally, physically, and emotionally. Yet much of the focus in today's society is on the baby's development. Your recovery and new reality are just as important as, if not more important than, those milestones your baby will be hitting. If you aren't well, it's difficult to care for your baby.

Twelve weeks, however, is not a magic number that indicates you've made it through postpartum. Focus on taking care of yourself and your baby and not on "bouncing back" or hitting certain milestones.

In this section, I'll walk you through physical recovery from birth as well as emotional and hormonal shifts you may experience. We'll talk about feeding and caring for your baby and reaching out for help when you need it. I will be focusing on what a typical recovery looks like, but additional medical needs can come up. If you have any concerns, always check with your doctor or midwife.

Note: Since the recovery and developmental timeline varies for each mother and baby, I encourage you to go ahead and read through this entire section, and then you can refer back to certain weeks for a refresher if needed.

Chapter 10

Baby's First Month

Newborn babies are so sweet and snuggly, and they will let you know, quite loudly, when they need something. I encourage you to follow the "sleep when baby sleeps" advice, at least during this first month. You're recovering from giving birth while caring for baby's every need; it's a lot!

First-Month Action Plan:

- Self-care and rest for you and your partner should be your number one priority after baby's needs are met.
- Some cultures honor a 40-day "lying-in" period during which Mom stays in bed and is completely taken care of so she can focus on baby. While 40 days in bed probably isn't feasible, I encourage you to accept help when offered.

First-Week Milestones

■ BABY'S STATS

+ Your baby will likely lose weight in the first two weeks of life, up to about 10 percent of their birth weight.
+ If breastfeeding remains painful for the duration of the feeding or your nipples are a lipstick shape when baby is done, you are likely getting a shallow latch and should talk to a lactation consultant.

■ MOM'S STATS

+ Your breasts can become engorged when your milk comes in around day 3 or 4 (though for some first-time moms, it can take longer). Feeding baby frequently is the best treatment.
+ You're likely experiencing heavy postpartum bleeding called lochia, along with some large clots. Generally, anything smaller than a golf ball is considered normal in the first few days. If you are soaking a maxi pad in less than an hour, tell your care provider.

■ NOT-TO-MISS APPOINTMENTS

If you've had a hospital birth, you will take your baby to the pediatrician around three to five days after birth. If you've had a birth-center birth or home birth, your midwife will probably visit you several times in the first couple of weeks to check on you and baby. The first visit is usually 24 to 48 hours after birth.

FIRST-WEEK GOALS

Symptoms 101 If you've had a vaginal birth, your vagina and perineum are likely sore and swollen, and you may be taking care of stitches and hemorrhoids. Use cold packs, stay horizontal as much as possible, and sit on an inflatable donut or Boppy pillow when you do have to sit up.

Rejuvenate Birthsong Botanicals makes a soothing postpartum herb bath, which was one of my favorite postpartum practices. My midwife advised me to take my baby into the bath for about 10 minutes, since the same herbs that are healing for your perineum also help dry up baby's umbilical cord. If you don't have time for a full bath, a sitz bath is a good substitute.

There is a drastic shift in hormones around day 4 or 5 after your milk comes in, and it can make you extremely emotional. Your progesterone and estrogen levels drop back to near-normal levels, but oxytocin and prolactin spike to support bonding and breastfeeding.

Between 70 and 80 percent of women will experience "baby blues" when this happens, which lasts about two weeks. You may be weepy and feel sad or irritable, but unlike the more serious conditions of PPD or PPA (page 100), you are also able to experience moments of joy. Getting extra sleep will often ease your symptoms.

Second-Week Milestones

■ BABY'S STATS

+ If you're breastfeeding, baby's poop will be basically liquid that is yellow and "seedy." If you're formula feeding, baby's poop will be similar to peanut butter. Yum!

+ Baby's umbilical cord is drying up and will likely fall off this week. If you notice it oozing pus or bleeding, talk to your care provider.

■ MOM'S STATS

+ Your postpartum bleeding should be decreasing and becoming dark brown versus bright red. You may still experience some blood clots, but they should be closer to the size of a quarter or smaller.
+ You're more sleep deprived than you've ever been in your life, and emotions can run high. Ask for help as much as you can.

■ NOT-TO-MISS APPOINTMENTS

Baby will have another checkup this week, and if you've had an out-of-hospital birth, your midwife will check on you as well. Most women who give birth in the hospital don't see their ob-gyn again until six weeks postpartum. A lot can happen in six weeks, so don't hesitate to make an appointment if something doesn't feel right physically or mentally.

SECOND-WEEK GOALS

Gear Up If your nipples are sore or cracking, apply cold gel packs or silver nipple soothers between feedings, and use a nipple balm before and after every feeding. A saltwater soak of 1 cup warm water with ½ teaspoon salt will help keep cracked nipples from getting infected. Fill two small glasses (shot glasses work well) and soak your nipples for about five minutes right after nursing.

Baby Care Try to catch early hunger cues from your baby, like stirring from sleep, opening their mouth, and rooting (bobbing or turning their head). If you've missed these cues, baby will start crying, thrashing, and turning red. Try to catch the early cues so you don't have to calm baby down before they are able to eat.

KEY ADVICE

Twenty-five percent of American mothers go back to work by 14 days postpartum. If this is you, my heart goes out to you. I could write a whole chapter on how insane it is that we don't require paid family leave in the United States, but it won't change the fact that you have to figure out how to continue to heal your body, work to pay your bills, and leave your baby in someone else's care. That being said, some states do offer paid family leave benefits, and you can sometimes combine multiple programs (e.g., short-term disability and paid family leave), so it's worth looking into your options.

Clogged Ducts and Mastitis

If you breastfeed and your baby isn't emptying your breasts effi-
ciently, or you have a large milk supply, or you just get a case of
bad luck, you might get a clogged duct. If a clogged duct becomes
infected, it causes mastitis. About 20 percent of new moms in the
United States will get mastitis, and it is most common in the first two
to three weeks.

If you have a clogged duct, you can often feel a hard wedge under
the skin and visibly see a swollen or hard area on your breast. Signs
of mastitis include flu-like symptoms, fever, and red streaks extend-
ing out from the affected duct.

You can still breastfeed, but you will need to get the clogged duct
to clear as well as see a doctor for an antibiotic prescription. You
should stay in bed as much as possible and nurse, nurse, nurse—at
least every two hours. Drink plenty of water and eat nutritious foods.
You can apply wet heat to the clogged duct and gently massage the
affected area in the direction toward your nipple. Some moms find
cold cabbage leaves and cold compresses relieve inflammation and
pain between feedings.

After you've recovered, it's normal for the affected breast to be
sore or even remain red for about a week.

Third-Week Milestones

■ BABY'S STATS

+ The goal is for baby to have gained back to their birth weight by the beginning of this week and to continue to gain about 6 ounces a week for the next few weeks.
+ Keep track of the number of diapers they wet and soil, aiming for about five to six wet diapers and three to four soiled diapers a day.

■ MOM'S STATS

+ If you had cracked and sore nipples, they should be close to healed by this week. Engorgement is also easing up.
+ Your uterus is shrinking, but you'll still want stretchy, comfy pants. Some women find a belly binder or girdle feels supportive.

■ NOT-TO-MISS APPOINTMENTS

If you had stiches, they should dissolve soon. Standard suture material takes four to six weeks to reabsorb. If you have any concerns about infection, be sure to consult your doctor or midwife. Continue taking herb baths or sitz baths if you're still experiencing discomfort.

THIRD-WEEK GOALS

Baby Care While feeding your baby, watch for jaw movement and listen for swallowing. If baby is falling asleep constantly, try getting them undressed, stroking their face, lifting their arm, and using breast compression if you're breastfeeding. This will often stimulate baby enough to nurse on your other breast or finish the bottle.

Rejuvenate Drink lots of water and eat a well-balanced diet filled with plenty of fruits and vegetables. Again, I love Heng Ou's book *The First Forty Days* for nutritious and healing recipes. If you are breastfeeding, it's recommended to get an extra 200 to 500 calories a day above your normal recommended caloric intake.

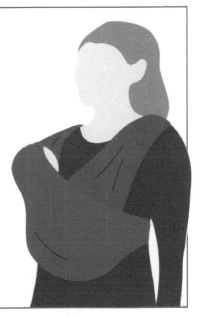

KEY ADVICE

Babywearing is a wonderful way to soothe a fussy baby and has the added benefit of freeing up your hands. Most cities have a babywearing group, where you can borrow a carrier and get a lesson on using it. Side note: Babywearing helps strengthen baby's neck and counts as "tummy time."

Fourth-Week Milestones

■ BABY'S STATS

+ Baby is gaining control of their muscles. You'll notice fewer jerky, reflexive movements.
+ Babies go through a growth spurt between four and six weeks and will want to eat more frequently.
+ If you are formula feeding, baby is likely increasing their intake from 2 to 3 ounces to at least 4 ounces every four hours. If you're breastfeeding, baby will be getting smaller amounts more frequently.

■ MOM'S STATS

You are likely starting to feel a little more balanced emotionally as your hormones continue to level out and you become accustomed to lack of sleep. It's normal to still have bouts of "baby blues," but if it's persistent, you may be experiencing one of the mood disorders we discussed on page 100.

■ NOT-TO-MISS APPOINTMENTS

Baby will likely have a one-month pediatrician appointment this week. Your pediatrician will ask how baby is sleeping, eating, and pooping. They will give baby a physical exam and look for developmental signs like focusing on objects and reacting to sounds. If your baby received a hepatitis B vaccine at birth, they will get their second dose at this appointment. If you had an out-of-hospital birth, you may continue to see your midwife until six weeks and then schedule your first pediatrician appointment.

FOURTH-WEEK GOALS

On the Menu If you're breastfeeding, your pediatrician will likely recommend that your baby get a vitamin D supplement. You can get liquid drops, and baby should get 400 IU a day. Alternatively, you can take a vitamin that contains at least 6400 IU of vitamin D, and evidence shows it will pass on to baby through your milk.

Baby Care You can begin "tummy time" with your baby to help them build their neck strength. This also helps prevent baby from getting a flat spot on the back of their head. If they seem like they hate this activity, try laying down on your back and putting them on your chest and singing to them or making silly sounds.

KEY ADVICE

If you're breastfeeding, now is the time to introduce a bottle to your baby. If you wait much longer than this, many babies will refuse a bottle. You should try to offer baby a bottle every other day to keep this skill up, although it doesn't need to be a whole bottle—even half an ounce is enough for them to practice.

Colic: What's All the Crying About?

Between 15 and 20 percent of babies will suffer from colic. Colic is not a medical diagnosis or condition, simply a term to describe a behavior. Doctors define colic as three or more straight hours of crying at least three days a week for at least three weeks (3-3-3). This can be extremely taxing on you, made worse by the fact that no one is exactly sure what causes colic, so it's hard to know how to handle it.

A few possible causes are digestive issues, low milk supply, environmental factors, and reflux or constant spitting up. The good news is that it usually goes away on its own as baby gets older (usually by three to four months of age), typically peaking around six weeks. While you wait it out, take turns caring for your baby with your partner or another helper, and ensure you're getting at least a few minutes throughout the day of quiet alone time.

A great resource for learning soothing techniques is Harvey Karp's *The Happiest Baby on the Block*. I also encourage you to look into the "Period of PURPLE Crying" at purplecrying.info for coping techniques. Some doctors recommend Cranial Fascial Therapy (CFT) to ease symptoms of colic and a host of other conditions, including tongue tie, inability to latch, constipation, and general fussiness.

If you're ever feeling too overwhelmed or frustrated to care for your baby, it's okay to set them down in a safe place, like their crib, and walk away for a few minutes until you are calm enough to pick them up again.

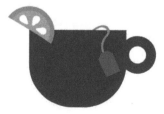

Chapter 11

Baby's Second Month

Can you believe your baby is already one month old? It really does fly by, and yet at the same time, it's hard to believe you've survived for a whole month on so little sleep. Month 2 comes with some major developmental changes for baby, and hopefully you're starting to get into a rhythm.

Second-Month Action Plan:

- Become familiar with baby's developmental leaps using Hetty van de Rijt and Frans Plooij's *The Wonder Weeks* book and/or app so you can anticipate sleep regressions and crankiness.
- Check in on your physical and emotional recovery and reach out for help if needed.

Fifth-Week Milestones

■ BABY'S STATS

+ Baby is entering their first developmental leap, which can mean a sleep regression and extra fussiness.
+ While they may be fussy, many babies also start to smile, on purpose, around this time.
+ Baby is still eating around 10 times a day and should be gaining about 5 to 7 ounces a week.

■ MOM'S STATS

+ Your postpartum bleeding should be minimal at this point. If you notice your bleeding going from brown or pink back to red, you are likely overdoing it and should rest more. If it continues to be heavy, you should consult your care provider.
+ You may start feeling ready for light exercise, and if the weather is cooperating, a little sunshine on a daily walk with baby can be great for your mood.

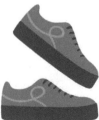

■ NOT-TO-MISS APPOINTMENTS

If you're experiencing any back or neck pain, make an appointment with a chiropractor. Giving birth can throw you out of alignment. Plus, breastfeeding often causes you to contort yourself in all kinds of crazy ways that can cause soreness.

FIFTH-WEEK GOALS

Career Coach If you're going back to work soon, check in with your supervisor and see whether you can adjust your schedule if needed, and make sure there is a place for you to pump if you're breastfeeding and plan to continue.

Baby Care In the United States, infant formula is regulated by the FDA, and all formulas are basically the same. The main thing to consider is whether your formula is dairy based, soy based, or protein hydrolysate (also called hypoallergenic). You may also want to consider organic or non-GMO options if that's important to you. The ready-to-feed liquid formula is sterile and generally considered safer for newborns than the powdered form. If you're using powdered formula, be sure you are following safe preparation guidelines and using filtered water. The CDC has guidelines on preparing infant formula at cdc.gov.

There are 10 mental leaps that all babies go through developmentally in the first 20 months of life. An amazing resource for understanding the mental leaps that your baby goes through is Hetty van de Rijt and Frans Plooij's book The Wonder Weeks. *They also have an app that will send you notifications and tips when your baby is about to enter another leap.*

Sixth-Week Milestones

■ BABY'S STATS

+ Baby is focusing on objects and may stare at something for quite a while. Ceiling fans are a favorite.
+ Many babies go through another growth spurt and may be extra fussy, but the good news is that after this week they will have passed the peak age for fussiness in general.

■ MOM'S STATS

Your uterus should have shrunk back down to the size of a fist, but that doesn't mean your tummy is back to "normal." Your skin and abdominal muscles may be forever changed by pregnancy.

■ NOT-TO-MISS APPOINTMENTS

You will have a final postpartum checkup this week with your ob-gyn or midwife. Your care provider will give you a pelvic exam to check your cervix and ovaries. They will also most likely give you a Pap smear and will look at your incision if you had a cesarean birth. This is also an ideal time to discuss birth control options.

SIXTH-WEEK GOALS

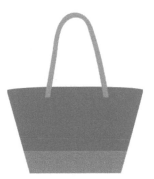

Gear Up If you're going back to work in the next few weeks, start to think about a feeding plan for baby. If you're breastfeeding, you'll want to have a couple of days' milk stash saved, but you don't need a freezer full. You'll want to pump enough at work to keep up with baby's demand so your milk supply doesn't decrease. *Work. Pump. Repeat.* by Jessica Shortall is a great book, and *The Birth Hour* has a Back-2-Work Breastfeeding class you can access at thebirthhour.com.

Rejuvenate Most people know about prenatal massage, but postpartum massage is equally wonderful. Many massage therapists offer house calls for new mothers and are flexible if you need to nurse your baby during your session.

You may have heard that the six-week mark is when you will be "cleared" for sex and exercise. I always assumed there was some biological reason for this, but it turns out there's no medical evidence for why this week is chosen. You may still not feel ready physically or emotionally for sex or exercise. Everybody heals differently, and it's common to have zero sex drive postpartum. Many women I've interviewed report that sex was still painful at 6 weeks, better closer to 12 weeks, but not truly enjoyable until close to a year postpartum. Don't feel pressured to meet any expectations set by this timeline.

Seventh-Week Milestones

■ BABY'S STATS

+ Baby is consuming between 18 and 36 ounces of milk a day, approximately every three hours. Remember, though, babies can't tell time, and you should try to feed on demand—especially if you're breastfeeding.

+ Baby is starting to differentiate between day and night, so you may get at least one longer nighttime stretch of sleep, possibly up to four to six hours.

■ MOM'S STATS

If you had a cesarean birth, your scar has healed but may feel numb or itchy. You should be cleared this week to lift objects heavier than your baby.

■ NOT-TO-MISS APPOINTMENTS

If you have a partner, or someone helping you, come up with a game plan to make sleep and self-care a priority for everyone. Maybe you take the early morning shift while your partner sleeps in, and then they take the fussy evening "witching hour" so you can take a long bath or get out of the house for a bit.

SEVENTH-WEEK GOALS

Baby Care Sometimes it seems like your baby is spitting up their entire feeding, but it's likely no more than a tablespoon. Babies are born without fully developed digestive systems, so this is normal. If baby is a "happy spitter," no need to worry. If they seem to be in a lot of pain or are arching their back, ask your doctor about reflux.

Gear Up There are so many adorable swaddle blankets, but, unfortunately, many babies become little Houdinis around this time and can wriggle their arms out. When your baby gets to this stage, I recommend the Miracle Blanket or Love to Dream Swaddle UP. Once baby starts rolling over, it's no longer safe to swaddle.

You may have noticed your baby's skin breaking out. Baby acne is due to the release of hormones baby received from you during pregnancy, so no topical treatment will alleviate it. The good news is that it usually clears up within a couple of weeks.

Eighth-Week Milestones

■ BABY'S STATS

+ Baby enters another mental leap this week and may be fussier than usual or sleep more or less than normal.
+ Baby weighs somewhere around 11 to 13 pounds and is between 22 and 23 inches long, with boys typically being bigger than girls.

■ MOM'S STATS

If you're exclusively breastfeeding, you may not get your period for quite a while, although for some women menstruation returns regardless of breastfeeding. Start considering contraception methods, even if your period hasn't returned, because you can ovulate prior to your first postpartum period and end up with a surprise sibling for your baby!

■ NOT-TO-MISS APPOINTMENTS

Baby will have a well-baby checkup this month. Baby will be weighed and measured, and you'll hear what percentile their growth is. The 50th percentile is the average, but the number doesn't really matter as long as your baby continues to grow at a proportional rate for them. The CDC recommends several vaccines at this appointment, so come prepared with any questions you have.

EIGHTH-WEEK GOALS

Baby Care Most babies poop a ton! Every time you hear them pass gas, you'll notice that they likely also pooped. It can be a little alarming when they go a day or more without pooping, but it's rare for a baby to be constipated, especially if you're breastfeeding.

Gear Up Speaking of all that poop, baby may get a diaper rash. The best medicine is prevention, so try to change soiled diapers as soon as they happen, and be sure that baby's bottom is completely dry before putting a new diaper on. If the rash won't clear up, consult your pediatrician. It could be a yeast infection that requires a prescription cream.

Diastasis recti is a gap in your abdominal muscles caused by your growing uterus during pregnancy. Ninety-eight percent of women have this at the end of pregnancy, but the gap should close by about eight weeks postpartum. This gap is usually, but not always, accompanied by a protruding stomach, and it can cause incontinence and other pelvic floor issues. To check whether you have diastasis recti, lie on your back, put your fingertips on your belly button, and lift your head like you're doing a small crunch to engage your abdominal muscles. Repeat this above and below your belly button as well. If you feel a gap that can fit two or more fingers, then you should seek help.

Chapter 12

Baby's Third Month

This is the final month that baby is considered a newborn. It's crazy how much baby's appearance changes during these months. Maybe baby looked just like Grandpa at birth, and now their features are completely different. The entire first year is full of growth and changes, both for baby and, maybe even more so, for you.

Third-Month Action Plan:

- Make a plan for returning to work, or not, and focus on what a healthy work/life balance will look like for your family.
- From this point on, baby is hitting developmental milestones at a rapid rate—refer to your Wonder Weeks app for ideas on how to help baby learn.

Ninth-Week Milestones

■ BABY'S STATS

It's truly remarkable what baby has learned in just two months of life. You are getting lots of smiles and maybe even the occasional laugh. A baby's laugh might be my favorite sound in the world!

■ MOM'S STATS

Some women notice acne appearing when they are breastfeeding or when they stop. As with most things pregnancy, this is related to hormonal shifts. You may want to consult a dermatologist, but it should clear up when your hormones level out.

■ NOT-TO-MISS APPOINTMENTS

You may start to feel ready to exercise over the next month. Start slow, with light walks or yoga. Joining a gym or YMCA is a great option because they typically offer childcare. Getting into the habit of working out is a lot easier when you know you'll get an hour or so of childcare. I recommend starting this before baby enters their separation-anxiety phase, usually around six to eight months.

NINTH-WEEK GOALS

Baby Care Talk to your baby as much as possible and wait for their response. I know they aren't much of a conversationalist, but hearing you talk will help them learn. Narrate what you're doing as you're doing it, even if it feels a little silly. It's amazing to watch baby listen and then coo in response.

Budget Boot Camp If you'll have childcare expenses, look into a dependent-care flexible spending account with your or your partner's employer. Your company can take money from your paycheck, pre-taxes, to cover childcare expenses. It can save you about 30 percent. Keep your childcare receipts, too, because everyone can take advantage of the dependent-care tax credit when filing tax returns.

■ BABY'S STATS

Baby is learning to self-soothe and may start to really like the pacifier or their thumb. Try a few different pacifiers, since each baby will have their own preferences.

■ MOM'S STATS

If you're breastfeeding and you start to notice that your breasts don't seem as full, don't immediately assume low milk supply is the issue. It's likely just your body adjusting to baby's demands. If baby is sleeping more, your milk supply will adjust to prevent engorgement.

■ NOT-TO-MISS APPOINTMENTS

Learn the ins and outs of safe milk storage. Freshly pumped breast milk can sit on the counter for up to four hours or in the refrigerator for two days. Prepared formula should not sit out at room temperature for more than an hour and should only be stored in the refrigerator for 24 hours. Premixed liquid formula can only be stored in the refrigerator for two days after being opened.

TENTH-WEEK GOALS

Gear Up Download an app to record feedings, sleep, and diaper changes so you have one less thing to think about. This can also come in handy when you are sharing baby duty with your partner or another caretaker. Ovia Parenting is a great, free option.

Baby Care If you've been breastfeeding but want to start supplementing with formula or pumped milk, consider using the lowest flow nipple, or even a preemie nipple, so that baby doesn't get used to the faster flow that bottles provide. This is also a great tip for formula-fed babies to prevent overfeeding.

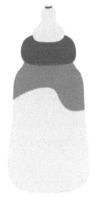

> ### KEY ADVICE
>
> *The phrase "bounce back" is pretty silly, as there really is no going back after having a baby, only forward. All postpartum bodies recover differently, and being prepared for your belly, hips, breasts, and skin to look, well, different, can go a long way. Your body just did this completely amazing thing—growing and birthing a human. The remaining physical evidence of that accomplishment is part of your story as a mother.*

Eleventh-Week Milestones

■ BABY'S STATS

+ Baby is about to enter another growth spurt and may want to "cluster feed," which basically just means eat all the time.
+ Baby will anticipate you picking them up and may get all four limbs going like an adorable beetle on its back to let you know they are ready for you!

■ MOM'S STATS

You may notice an emotional shift where you feel somewhat alone. The visitors aren't coming any more. If you have a partner, they have returned to their normal work schedule, and you're at home every day with the baby. These feelings are common, but if you notice that you're sad or anxious all the time, review those signs of PPD and PPA on page 100. These mood disorders can show up any time during the first year.

■ NOT-TO-MISS APPOINTMENTS

If you're going back to work soon, consider a trip to your workplace to get your things organized and make sure there is a place to pump and store your milk if you plan to continue breastfeeding. You can sneak in on the weekend or go during the week and introduce your coworkers to your baby.

ELEVENTH-WEEK GOALS

Baby Care If your baby suddenly won't take stashed breast milk, it could have excess lipase, an enzyme that breaks down the fats in breast milk and creates a sour or soapy taste. There is a method of scalding your milk that you can follow in order to save it. I recommend exclusivepumping.com for instructions on how to do this.

Gear Up Even though baby isn't mobile yet, it can't hurt to start thinking about babyproofing your home. I swear, babies are mesmerized by wall outlets and will roll over to them well before they start crawling. Other things to consider are anchoring heavy furniture to the wall and adding childproof latches to your cabinets.

KEY ADVICE

If you're getting out and about more, you're likely answering lots of questions, and everyone will want to know whether baby is a "good sleeper" and whether they are sleeping through the night. Keep in mind that a five-hour stretch of sleep is considered sleeping through the night for babies this age.

Twelfth-Week Milestones

■ BABY'S STATS

Baby can roll from side to side and may even be able to roll from their tummy to their back.

■ MOM'S STATS

Your hair may begin to fall out sometime in the next couple of months. This is due to hormonal changes, and it can seem like you're losing A LOT! Don't worry, you aren't going to go bald, and it is growing back in at the same time. You'll start to notice a lot of little baby hairs around your hairline.

■ NOT-TO-MISS APPOINTMENTS

Baby isn't on much of a schedule yet, but it's never too early to create a soothing sleep environment and begin sleep associations. A study in 2008 showed that having a fan going in baby's room reduced the risk of SIDS by 70 percent, a statistic worthy of a trip to the store! As far as sleep associations, some ideas include a bath, reading a book, singing a song, and zipping baby into a sleep sack, or swaddling if they aren't rolling over yet.

TWELFTH-WEEK GOALS

Career Coach If you plan to work from home, you likely still need help. Babies are unpredictable at this age, so it's hard to schedule work around their naps, or lack thereof. Try to find at least a few hours of childcare each day. Sometimes a mother's helper is more affordable than a nanny since you're home to help if needed.

Rejuvenate Lack of sleep can make everything seem more intense. If you or your partner are feeling defeated, a nap or good night's sleep can go a long way. Once baby gets into more of a routine, try to put them to bed no later than 8 p.m.

KEY ADVICE

If you're going back to work next week (or already have), I know there's a lot on your mind. You might be dreading leaving your baby, or maybe you're excited to see your work friends and use your brain again for non-baby-related things. Regardless, it's a big transition. For many moms, the first few days or weeks are hard and emotional. It will get easier, I promise.

If you've decided to stay home with your baby, create a routine and make regular plans to get out of the house so you don't feel isolated. Staying home with your baby is a big transition too!

The Days Are Long, but the Years Are Short

You've come a long way from getting that positive pregnancy test. You have accomplished so much over the last year, and it's worth taking a moment to revel in the superwoman that you are!

Now that you are coming out of the haze of newborn-hood, caring for your baby will start to feel more natural. But there will always be new challenges: From crawling, eating solids, teething, and preschool, to learning to drive and moving out, this parenthood gig is never-ending. For now, as you encounter new phases, remember to consult the research and evidence. But also lean into your intuition, which has become fine-tuned over the past year. Don't discount the mama instincts that come naturally to you.

The next 9 months will go by at the same rapid pace as the last 12. I view baby's first birthday as a celebration of *the parents* making it through year one. It's a lot to adjust to, and you are doing an amazing job. Now, take everything you've learned in this book and through your own experiences over the past year, and offer love and judgment-free support to your sister-in-law, or your best friend, or the mom struggling with her stroller trying to get on the airplane. Becoming a mother opens your eyes to just how hard a job it really is. The best thing you can do with this new-found knowledge is find the support you deserve and then pay it forward.

References

Academy of Breastfeeding Medicine Protocol Committee. 2008.
"ABM Clinical Protocol #6: Guideline on Co-sleeping and Breastfeeding: Revision, March 2008." *Breastfeeding Medicine* 3 (1):
38–43. doi:10.1089/bfm.2007.9979.

Amato, Paula, and Maggie Blott, eds. 2018. *Pregnancy Day by
Day: Count Down Your Pregnancy Day by Day with Advice from
a Team of Experts and Amazing Images for Every Stage of Your
Baby's Development.* New York: DK.

American Academy of Pediatrics. 2012. "Circumcision
Policy Statement." *Pediatrics* 130 (3): 585-86. doi:10.1542
/peds.2012–1989.

American Academy of Pediatrics. 2019. "Safe Sleep." Accessed
July 2, 2019. https://www.aap.org/en-us/advocacy-and
-policy/aap-health-initiatives/child_death_review/Pages
/Safe-Sleep.aspx.

American College of Obstetricians and Gynecologists. 2017.
"When Pregnancy Goes Past Your Due Date." Accessed June 29,
2019. https://www.acog.org/Patients/FAQs/When-Pregnancy
-Goes-Past-Your-Due-Date.

American College of Obstetricians and Gynecologists
Committee on Obstetric Practice. 2017. "Committee Opinion
Number 684: Delayed Umbilical Cord Clamping after Birth."
Obstetrics and Gynecology 129 (1): e5–e10. doi:10.1097/aog
.0000000000001860.

American Pregnancy Association. 2019. "Miscarriage: Signs, Symptoms, Treatment, and Prevention." Accessed June 16, 2019. https://americanpregnancy.org/pregnancy-complications /miscarriage/.

The Birth Hour. 2019. "Essential Oils for Pregnancy: What Oils to Use and Avoid." Accessed June 26, 2019. https://thebirthhour .com/essential-oils-for-pregnancy-what-to-use-and-avoid -how-to-apply/.

Brody, Lauren Smith. 2018. *The Fifth Trimester: The Working Mom's Guide to Style, Sanity, and Success after Baby.* New York: Anchor Books.

Centers for Disease Control and Prevention. 2019. "Breastfeeding." Accessed June 30, 2019. https://www.cdc.gov/breastfeeding/.

Centers for Disease Control and Prevention. 2019. "Immuniza-tion Schedules." Accessed July 8, 2019. https://www.cdc.gov /vaccines/schedules/index.html.

Coleman-Phox, Kimberly, Roxana Odouli, and De-Kun Li. 2008. "Use of a Fan during Sleep and the Risk of Sudden Infant Death Syndrome." *Archives of Pediatrics and Adolescent Medicine* 162 (10): 963-68. doi:10.1001/archpedi.162.10.963.

Dekker, Rebecca. 2016. "Evidence On: Induction or C-section for a Big Baby?" *Evidence Based Birth.* Accessed June 16, 2019. https://evidencebasedbirth.com/evidence-for-induction-or-c -section-for-big-baby/.

Dekker, Rebecca. 2017. "The Evidence On: Group B Strep." *Evidence Based Birth.* Accessed June 22, 2019. https://evidencebasedbirth.com/groupbstrep/.

Deshpande, Parijat. 2018. *Pregnancy Brain: A Mind-Body Approach to Stress Management during a High-Risk Pregnancy.* Parijat Deshpande, LLC.

Gaskin, Ina May. 2003. *Ina May's Guide to Childbirth.* New York: Bantam Books.

Harshe, January. 2019. *Birth without Fear: The Judgment-Free Guide to Taking Charge of Your Pregnancy, Birth, and Postpartum.* New York: Hatchette.

HealthCare.gov. 2019. "Breastfeeding Benefits." Accessed June 29, 2019. https://www.healthcare.gov/coverage/breast -feeding-benefits/.

Hoffman, Benjamin D., Adrienne R. Gallardo, and Kathleen F. Carlson. 2016. "Unsafe from the Start: Serious Misuse of Car Safety Seats at Newborn Discharge." *Journal of Pediatrics* 171: 48–54. doi:10.1016/j.jpeds.2015.11.047.

Karp, Harvey. 2015. *The Happiest Baby on the Block: The New Way to Calm Crying and Help Your Newborn Baby Sleep Longer.* 2nd ed. New York: Bantam Books.

Kondo, Marie. 2014. *The Life-Changing Magic of Tidying Up: The Japanese Art of Decluttering and Organizing.* Translated by Cathy Hirano. Berkeley, CA: Ten Speed Press.

Lukes, Casie Leigh. 2019. "The Truth about Postpartum Hormones and Healing: A Q&A with Aviva Romm, MD." *Experience Life.* Accessed June 30, 2019. https://experiencelife.com/article /postpartum-hormones/.

National Center on Shaken Baby Syndrome. 2019. "The Period of PURPLE Crying." Accessed July 3, 2019. http://www .purplecrying.info/.

Oster, Emily. 2014. *Expecting Better: Why the Conventional Pregnancy Wisdom Is Wrong—and What You Really Need to Know*. New York: Penguin.

Oster, Emily. 2019. *Cribsheet: A Data-Driven Guide to Better, More Relaxed Parenting, from Birth to Preschool*. New York: Penguin.

Ou, Heng. 2016. *The First Forty Days: The Essential Art of Nourishing the New Mother*. New York: Stewart, Tabori and Chang.

Sears, Wiliam, and Martha Sears. 2013. *The Healthy Pregnancy Book: Month by Month, Everything You Need to Know from America's Baby Experts*. With Linda Holt and B. J. Snell. Sears Parenting Library. New York: Little, Brown.

Shortall, Jessica. 2015. *Work. Pump. Repeat.: The New Mom's Survival Guide to Breastfeeding and Going Back to Work*. New York: Harry N. Abrams.

U.S. Department of Labor. 2019. "Family and Medical Leave (FMLA)." Accessed July 6, 2019. https://www.dol.gov/general/topic/benefits-leave/fmla.

Van de Rijt, Hetty, and Frans Plooij. 2017. *The Wonder Weeks: How to Stimulate the Most Important Development Weeks in Your Baby's First 20 Months and Turn These 10 Predictable, Great, Fussy Phases into Magical Leaps Forward*. 5th ed. With Xaviera Plas-Plooij. Arnhem, Netherlands: Kiddy World Publishing.

World Health Organization Human Reproduction Programme. 2015. "WHO Statement on Caesarean Section Rates." *Reproductive Health Matters* 23 (45): 149-50. doi:10.1016/j.rhm.2015.07.007.

Resources

Pregnancy

Medications during pregnancy: mothertobaby.org
Plus-size pregnancy: plussizebirth.com and sizefriendly.com
Twins and multiples: twiniversity.com
Find a chiropractor: icpa4kids.com
Baby positioning: spinningbabies.com
Essential oils in pregnancy: thebirthhour.com/essential-oils

Pregnancy Loss Support

Still Standing Magazine: stillstandingmag.com
Pregnancy after Loss Support (PALS): pregnancyafterloss
support.com
@ihadamiscarriage Instagram Account

Birth

Listen to birth stories: thebirthhour.com/birth-stories
Find a doula: doulamatch.net or dona.org
Compare hospitals and view statistics: leapfroggroup.org
or babyfriendlyusa.org
International Cesarean Awareness Network: ican-online.org
Vaginal birth after cesarean: vbacfacts.com
Vaginal breech delivery: informedpregnancy.com/heads-up
Birthing instincts: birthinginstincts.com

Evidence Based Birth: evidencebasedbirth.com

Cord blood donation: bethematch.org

Premature infants: marchofdimes.org and grahams foundation.org

Childbirth Methodologies and Education

The Birth Hour's Know Your Options online course: thebirthhour.com

Lamaze International: lamaze.org

The Bradley Method: bradleybirth.com

HypnoBirthing: us.hypnobirthing.com

Birthing from Within: birthingfromwithin.com

Breastfeeding Support

Breast milk donation: Human Milk for Human Babies local Facebook groups

La Leche League International: llli.org

Help getting breast pump through insurance: aeroflowbreastpumps.com

Find a lactation consultant: ilca.org or uslca.org

Evidence-based information on breastfeeding: kellymom.com

Pumping information: exclusivepumping.com

The Birth Hour's Back-2-Work Breastfeeding online course: thebirthhour.com

Postpartum Support and Recovery

Postpartum Progress: postpartumprogress.com

Postpartum support 24/7 hotline: postpartum.net

Diastasis recti and pelvic floor recovery: mutusystem.com

Baby

Universal baby registry: babylist.com

Infant CPR class: redcross.org

Organize meals from friends: mealtrain.com

Car seat installation: safekids.org or thetotsquad.com

Babywearing tips and meetups: babywearinginternational.org

Newborn sleep tips and online course: takingcarababies.com

Smartphone Apps

Ovia: keep track of everything from fertility to pregnancy and beyond

The Wonder Weeks: baby's developmental leaps

Expectful: pregnancy and postpartum guided meditation

Breastfeeding Solutions: help with common breastfeeding issues

LactMed: database of drugs and supplements that may have effects on a nursing baby and alternative options to consider

Index

Acknowledgments

My heartfelt gratitude to the incredibly hardworking team at Callisto Media, most especially Myryah Irby and Sara Kendall, for helping this book come together.

Thank you to Stephanie Spitzer-Hanks, my partner in creating the Know Your Options online childbirth course, for your commitment to delivering evidence-based information to our students in the most compassionate way. I'm constantly learning from you and so grateful the "birth world" brought us together.

I cannot begin to fully express my thanks to those who share their stories on *The Birth Hour* and the listeners who receive them with open arms, free of judgment. Without your support, none of this would have ever been possible. An extra special thanks to my listener-supporters' Patreon group for being a sounding board throughout the writing process.

I have been lucky enough to have many wonderful friendships throughout my life. To those who have influenced and encouraged me, from childhood through motherhood—y'all know who you are, and I thank you sincerely for your friendship.

Thank you to my parents for instilling in me the belief that I could do anything I set my mind to and for never putting a limit on the number of books on my shelf.

To Adelaide, Darwin, and Harvey: Your births showed me my greatest strength and are the defining moments of my life. Being your mama has opened my heart and mind in ways I never could have imagined. My love for you is boundless, and watching you grow and discover who you are in this world is the ultimate gift.

Most importantly, to Richard—my compass, best friend, and partner in life and parenthood—thank you for absolutely everything. You've always supported my dreams, even when I wasn't quite sure of them myself. Your love, patience, and many weekends taking the kids on adventures so I can work mean everything to me. Oh, and I love you more.

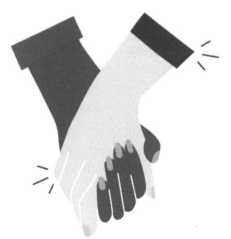

About the Author

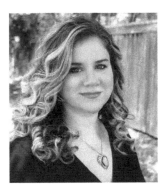 **Bryn Huntpalmer** is the founder of *The Birth Hour* podcast, which has been featured on the front page of Apple Podcasts and has over eight million downloads to date. She is passionate about helping women prepare for childbirth through the sharing of empowering and informative birth stories as well as *The Birth Hour*'s online, evidence-based childbirth course, Know Your Options.

She lives in Austin, Texas, with her husband, Richard, and their three kids, Harvey, Darwin, and Adelaide. She considers it her most important job to raise her children to be kind, aware, and courageous human beings.

Find Bryn at TheBirthHour.com or on social media @TheBirthHour.

CPSIA information can be obtained
at www.ICGtesting.com
Printed in the USA
BVHW061254061219
565760BV00002B/2/P